30 DAYS

- OF -

SEX TALKS

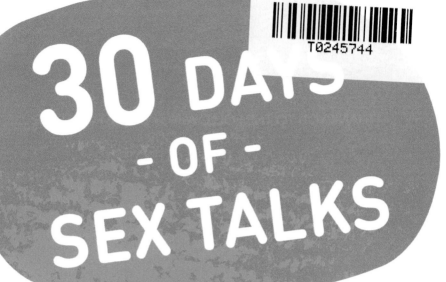

FOR LATTER-DAY SAINT FAMILIES

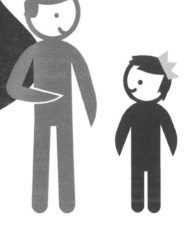

AGES
8–11

EMPOWERING YOUR CHILD WITH
KNOWLEDGE OF SEXUAL INTIMACY

IF YOU ENJOYED THIS BOOK,

PLEASE LEAVE A POSITIVE REVIEW ON

AMAZON.COM

THANK YOU TO THE FOLLOWING PEOPLE FOR THEIR
SUPPORT OF OUR
30 DAYS OF SEX TALKS PROJECTS

ED ALLISON

MARY ANN BENSON, MSW, LSW

SCOTT HOUNSELL

CLIFF PARK

Educate and Empower Kids, LLC
© 2024 by Educate and Empower Kids
All rights reserved.

This is not an official publication of the Church of Jesus Christ of Latter-day Saints. The opinions and views expressed herein belong solely to the author and do not necessarily represent the opinions or views of Cedar Fort, Inc. Permission for the use of sources, graphics, and photos is also solely the responsibility of the author.

ISBN 13: 978-1-4621-4617-8

Published by CFI, an imprint of Cedar Fort, Inc.
2373 W. 700 S., Suite 100, Springville, UT 84663
Distributed by Cedar Fort, Inc., www.cedarfort.com

Library of Congress Control Number: 2024936331

Cover design by Shawnda T. Craig
Cover design © 2024 Cedar Fort, Inc.

Printed in the United States of America

10 9 8 7 6 5 4 3 2 1

Printed on acid-free paper

For great resources and information, follow us:

Facebook: www.facebook.com/lds.eduempowerkids
Pinterest: @EmpowerLDSKids
Instagram: @eduempowerkids and @latterdaysaintkids
www.educateempowerkids.org
www.empowerlatterdaysaintkids.org

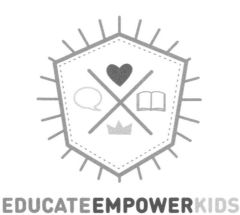

EDUCATE**EMPOWER**KIDS

Educate and Empower Kids would like to acknowledge the following people who contributed time, talents, and energy to this publication:

Dina Alexander, MS
Jenny Webb, MA
Amanda Scott
Caron C. Andrews

K. Parker
Trishia Van Orden
Fiona Leikness
Tina Mattsson-Bonett

Design and Illustration by:
Jera Mehrdad and Zachary Hourigan

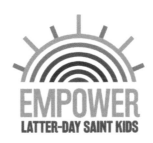

EMPOWER
LATTER-DAY SAINT KIDS

30 DAYS
- OF -
SEX TALKS

AGES
8–11

FOR LATTER-DAY
SAINT FAMILIES

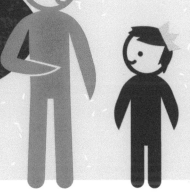

EMPOWERING YOUR CHILD WITH
KNOWLEDGE OF SEXUAL INTIMACY

CFI • AN IMPRINT OF CEDAR FORT, INC.
SPRINGVILLE, UTAH

30 DAYS OF SEX TALKS
FOR LATTER-DAY SAINT FAMILIES

• CONTENTS TOPICS FOR AGES 8–11 •

"We cannot wait for conversion to simply happen to our children. Accidental conversion is not a principle of the gospel of Jesus Christ. Becoming like our Savior will not happen randomly."

—Joy D. Jones

INTRODUCTION

Dear Parents and Guardians,

You and I both know that the most important work we will ever do on earth is to teach our children to be good, valiant, covenant-keeping people. Our homes are the first and most important schoolroom our children will have. This makes it the perfect place to have deep, meaningful conversations about important topics like love, healthy relationships, celestial marriage, sexual intimacy, and the dangers that threaten their future happiness.

We are living in complicated and uncertain times. Our kids are surrounded by unhealthy or false messages about their bodies, relationships, and human sexuality. It is our job to teach them what is true and what is not. It is vital that we begin these discussions to help them understand what healthy sexuality is, how special their bodies are, their primary identity as children of God, AND that they can come to us as parents to find answers to questions.

"The Family: A Proclamation to the World" reminds us that, "Parents have a sacred duty to rear their children in love and righteousness, to provide for their physical and spiritual needs, and to teach them to love and serve one another, to observe the commandments of God, and be law-abiding citizens wherever they live." With this pragmatic, gospel-focused program, you will find many opportunities to start conversations about these essential topics. In addition, using these lessons will help you create an environment in your home which encourages open discussions about many other topics that come up as you are raising your child.

WHAT'S INCLUDED

This curriculum includes helpful directions, 30 simple, yet meaningful lessons, and an extensive glossary of over 130 terms to help you. Each lesson includes introductory points to consider, critical teaching information, scripture, powerful discussion questions, and additional resources to enrich your family's learning experience. Some topics even have an accompanying activity or song to inspire further conversation.

> If you are positive and real with your child when it comes to talking about sexual intimacy, they will learn that you are available not just for this conversation, but for ANY discussion.

PREPARING FOR SUCCESS

- Consider your individual child's age, developmental stage, and personality in conjunction with each topic, as well as your family's values and individual situation. These will help you adapt the material in order to produce the best discussion. It's important that you begin your daily talks with just one topic in mind and that you make every experience, however brief, truly meaningful.

- If you feel like your child isn't ready to discuss the details of each topic or if you feel that your child's knowledge is more advanced, please note that it is important to discuss things with your child based on their own maturity level; progressing or referring back at your own pace.

- Plan ahead of time but don't create an event. Having a plan or planning ahead of time will remove much of the awkwardness you might feel in talking about these subjects with your child. In not creating an event, you are making the discussions feel more spontaneous, the experience more repeatable, and yourself more approachable.

- Please know, you do not need not be an expert to have purposeful, informative discussions with your kids. In fact, we feel strongly that leaning on your own personal experiences—both mistakes and successes—is a great way to use life lessons to teach your child. If done properly, these talks will bring you closer to your child than you could have ever imagined.

- You know and love your child more than anyone, so you decide when and where these discussions take place. In time, you will recognize and enjoy teaching moments in everyday life with your child.

NEED TO KNOW

- This program is meant to be simple! It's organized into simple topics with bullet points to be straightforward and create conversations. Each lesson may only take 10 minutes, but allow more time for your kids' questions and extra family discussion.

- This curriculum is not a one-discussion-fits-all. You guide the conversation and lead the discussion according to your unique situation. If you have three children, you will likely have three different conversations about the same topic.

- No program can cover all aspects of sexual intimacy perfectly for every individual circumstance. You can empower yourself with the knowledge you gain from this program to share with your child what you feel is the most important.

INSTRUCTIONS

BE POSITIVE

Take the fear and shame out of these discussions. Sex is natural and wondrous, and your child should feel nothing but positivity about it from you. If you do feel awkward, stay calm and use matter-of-fact tones in your discussions. It's easier than you think—just open your mouth and begin! It will get easier with every talk you have. Even after just a few talks, both you and your child will begin to look forward to this time you are spending together. Use experiences from your own life to begin a discussion if it makes you feel more comfortable. We have listed some tough topics here, but they are all discussed in a positive, informative way. Don't worry, you've got this!

ANSWER YOUR CHILD'S QUESTIONS

> Taking the time to talk about these topics will reiterate to your child how important they are to you.

If you are embarrassed by your child's curiosity and questions, you're implying that there is something shameful about these topics. However, if you can answer those questions calmly and honestly, you're demonstrating that sexuality is positive, and that healthy relationships are something to look forward to when the time is right. Be sure to answer your child's questions practically and cheerfully, and your child will learn that you are available not just for this discussion, but for any discussion. It's okay if you don't have all the answers. Tell them you will look for the answers and get back to them.

FOCUS ON INTIMACY

Help your child understand how incredible and uniting sex can be. Don't just talk about the mechanics of sex. Spend a significant amount of time talking about the beauty of love, sex, and the reality of human relationships, how they are built and maintained. Children are constantly exposed to unhealthy examples of relationships in the media. Many examples in the media are teaching your child lessons about sexuality and interactions between people that are misleading, incomplete, or purely unhealthy. Real emotional intimacy is rarely portrayed. It's your job to teach and model what true intimacy actually is. Your child needs you to help connect the dots between healthy relationships and sexuality. Model positive ways for your child to care for and appreciate his or her body, and how to protect, have a positive attitude toward, and make favorable choices for that body.

BE THE SOURCE

Remember, you direct the conversations. Bring up the lesson points and questions that you feel are most important and allow the conversation to flow from there. You love and know your child better than anyone else, so you are the best person to judge what will be most effective. Pause and take into account your personal values, religious beliefs, individual personalities, and family dynamics. You, the parent, can and should be the best source of information about sex and intimacy for your child. If you don't discuss these topics, your child will look for answers from other, less reliable and sometimes harmful sources like the internet, various media, and other kids.

> You love and know your child better than anyone else, so you are the best person to judge what will be most effective.

Feel free to begin these talks with a prayer to ensure that the Spirit can attend you during these important discussions. The Bible Dictionary reminds us that "Prayer is the act by which the will of the Father and the will of the child are brought into correspondence with each other."

Never underestimate the power and influence you have with your children! They need you and they need your wisdom.

—Dina Alexander
Educate and Empower Kids

LET'S GET STARTED!

What a fun age this is! It is within this age group that children become much more aware of their bodies, the opposite gender, and the world around them. Knowledge about how the human body works, how your child's body is going to change, and how they can be ready for these changes will empower them. This age is also when children begin to have feelings of self-consciousness, being attracted to others, and general awareness of sexuality. This is why it's important to discuss relationships, body image, media, gender, masturbation, pornography, and protective information as well.

Remember, this program is meant to inspire conversations that assist you in fostering an environment where difficult discussions are made easier. Enjoy this time with your kids and take advantage of the one-on-one time these conversations facilitate. In time, you will become more comfortable talking about these topics with your child, and your bond will be strengthened.

1. PUBLIC VS. PRIVATE

Home should be a safe place where children are able to talk to their parents about any questions they might have. Start these conversations by having your children ask their questions (whether they're about sex or other topics). Discuss the Safe Zone mentioned in the introduction and remind your kids that they can ask you any question at any time, even ones that they think are strange, private, embarrassing, or "bad."

Parents typically discuss various aspects of spirituality or sexuality with their children at different ages. Help your kids understand that there's new information every child needs to hear at different stages in his or her life.

> **Public:**
> *Belonging to or for the use of all people in a specific area, or all people as a whole. Something that is public is common, shared, collective, communal, and widespread.*

Start the Conversation

Explain to your child that their siblings or friends may not be ready to discuss topics like sex and puberty, and that those topics should only be discussed with parents to avoid confusion. Make sure to explain your reasons for making these conversations private. A few examples are that some people are uncomfortable talking about sex, small children are at a different level of understanding, and are not ready to hear this yet, and sex isn't something to be discussed amongst children.

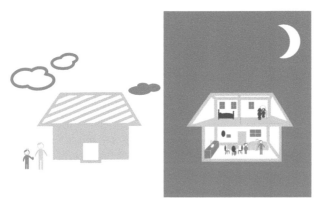

Discuss various times when it is appropriate to keep one's thoughts and comments to oneself, as well as when it's fitting to share spiritual experiences and stories. Make mention that our patriarchal blessings and temple ordinances are private, and talk about why sacred and special things should be kept private.

Questions for Your Child

- Why are some topics private? Why don't we talk about certain topics in public?

- Is it okay for an adult other than your parents to discuss sex with you?

- What are things we can talk about in public with our friends?

- What are some other topics that we consider public information?

> "Therefore, go ye unto your homes, and ponder upon the things which I have said, and ask of the Father, in my name, that ye may understand, and prepare your minds for the morrow, and I come unto you again."
>
> —3 Nephi 17:3

- Note: This is a great time to discuss internet use and what information we can publicly share vs. what information isn't safe to share. Consider talking about each of the following: Full name, school, address, religion, hobbies, phone number, medical history, location, grades, parent's location, income, interests, etc.

- What information is private and shouldn't be shared?

- Note: At this age, it is important to not only focus on activities one does in private but also conversations one has. We speak privately about sex, medical issues, and sacred experiences or beliefs, while we may talk about school, friends, and hobbies openly.

- Who should you discuss important private matters with?

- Have you and your friends ever talked about sex?

- Why is it not a good idea to talk to other kids about sex?

Additional Resources:

"I Need to Talk" from the *Friend*, April 2016
This is a great resource for helping children learn to talk about private things with a trusted adult.

"Bodily Integrity: Teaching Your Child to Make the Best Choices for His or Her Body" from Educate and Empower Kids
This article offers parents a variety of tips on how they can teach their children to love and respect their own bodies in a culture that would demand otherwise.

"Modesty and Smart Clothing Choices: Teaching Our Kids to Be Seen for Who They Are" from Educate and Empower Kids
This article helps to educate kids on what modesty means so that they're able to make smart, context-appropriate clothing choices that will empower them through a combination of self-respect and self-confidence.

2. MALE ANATOMY

Boys are created in the image of their Heavenly Father, just as girls are created in the image of their Heavenly Mother. Our heavenly parents formed our spirits long before we received our bodies. In creating our bodies, they gave us distinct and necessary differences. They also blessed us with many similarities.

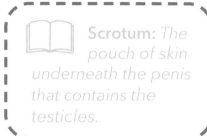

Scrotum: *The pouch of skin underneath the penis that contains the testicles.*

Use the glossary to help you discuss male anatomy (penis, testicle/scrotum, anus) with your child.

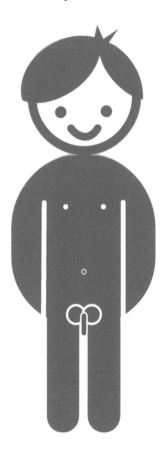

Start the Conversation

Teach your child that sexual organs are the most fundamental way that boys and girls are different. Explain that a doctor or nurse can look at a baby and know the sex of a baby. Discuss the purpose of the penis and scrotum—urination and ejaculation of sperm. (See the glossary for terms and explanations.) Explain how the penis and scrotum can expand and contract with body temperature. Feel free to discuss foreskin, circumcision, and your decision to circumcise or not.

If you have a diagram, now is a good time to use it. Talk about the breasts, nipples, and how, even in men, they can be tender. Describe how nipples can be many shapes, sizes, and colors. Asking your child if they have heard any slang terms is a good way to gauge if they have been talking about or hearing about sex outside your home.

Questions for Your Child

- What are some things that make boys and girls physically different?
- Why did God make us different?
- What similarities did God give us?
- What parts do you have? What parts does the opposite sex have?
- Men and women need each other! How do men and women compliment each other physically, spiritually, and emotionally?
- We have talked about the medically correct terms for these body parts, but there are many slang terms as well. What are some you have heard?
- People sometimes make jokes about body parts, especially our sex organs. This is the wrong attitude to have towards our bodies. Why are our sex organs special and private?

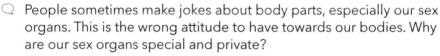

"In the image of his own body, male and female, created he them, and blessed them, and called their name Adam, in the day when they were created and became living souls in the land upon the footstool of God."

–Moses 6:9

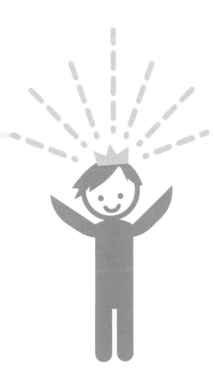

Additional Resources:

The Family: A Proclamation to the World
"All human beings—male and female—are created in the image of God. Each is a beloved spirit son or daughter of heavenly parents, and, as such, each has a divine nature and destiny."

"My Body- A Temple" from the *Friend*, May 2002
This piece discusses ways that we can treat our bodies and how to keep them clean. You can also make a little puppet that exercises.

Aaronic Priesthood Theme
"I am a beloved son of God, and He has a work for me to do."

3. FEMALE ANATOMY

Family night is a great time to talk about the uniqueness of boys and girls. Explain that girls are created in the image of their Heavenly Mother, just as boys are created in the image of Heavenly Father. Use "The Family: A Proclamation to the World" to discuss the necessity and blessing of having both men and

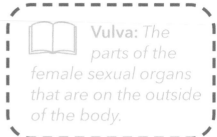

Vulva: *The parts of the female sexual organs that are on the outside of the body.*

women on earth. Feel free to quote the proclamation, "Gender is an essential characteristic of individual premortal, mortal, and eternal identity and purpose."

Use the glossary to help you discuss female anatomy (vagina, urethra, anus, breasts/nipples, vulva).

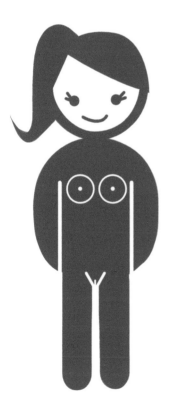

Start the Conversation

Discuss the many parts of the vagina and their functions. If you have a diagram, now is a good time to use it. If you are discussing this topic with your daughter, you may even want to encourage her to look at her vagina in a mirror. It is important for her to know exactly what it looks like and how it works. Remind her that every part of her body is special.

Describe how the anus is located in the same general area but is completely different from the vagina and is not a sexual organ. Talk about the purpose of breasts and nipples. Describe how they can be many shapes, sizes, and colors. Explain the many parts and uses of the vagina. See the glossary for additional definitions.

Questions for Your Child

○ What are some physical differences God gave boys and girls? What similarities did God give us?

○ Why do you think our heavenly parents sent both boys and girls to earth? Why are both needed?

○ We have talked about the medical terms for these body parts, but there are many slang terms as well. What are some you have heard?

○ What questions do you have about your body or how certain body parts work?

○ Every part of your body is special and worth protecting. Why do you think yours is worth protecting?

"So God created man in his own image, in the image of God created he him; male and female created he them."

–Genesis 1:27

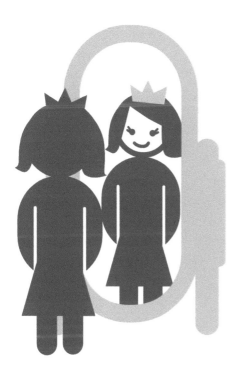

Additional Resources:

"Special Witness: Our Bodies Are Temples, and the Spirit of the Lord Should Dwell There and Shine Through" from the Friend, June 2008
"Our personal temples must be used to accomplish righteous purposes. Our physical body is a blessing, a timeless trust, and makes a forever family possible." –David A. Bednar

"Your Body: A Magnificent Gift to Cherish" from the *New Era*, August 2019
"May we ever be grateful for the incredible blessing of a magnificent physical body, the supreme creation of our loving Heavenly Father. As great as our body is, it is not an end in itself. It is an essential part of God's great plan of happiness for our eternal progression." –Russell M. Nelson

"Young Women Theme"
"I am a beloved daughter of heavenly parents, with a divine nature and eternal destiny."

4. PUBERTY FOR BOYS

Kids can sometimes freak out over puberty. For many, it can be scary going through physical changes that they have no control over. In a positive, encouraging manner, discuss the physical changes your son can expect: hair growth, more sweat, voice changes, etc. Explain the emotional changes too, due to increased hormone levels.

Don't forget to mention future adventures such as nocturnal emissions ("wet dreams") and spontaneous erections.

Nocturnal Emissions: *A spontaneous orgasm that occurs during sleep.*

Start the Conversation

Describe how boys begin to grow hair under their arms, in the pubic area, and will experience thicker growth in places like legs and arms and chest. Sweat glands will produce more sweat, and the area under the arms might smell unpleasant. The nipple and breast area may become tender and swell a bit. The voice will begin to deepen, and as a result, may "crack" occasionally. Touch on how emotional and sensitive boys can become during this time due to hormonal changes.

If you are discussing this with your son and he is ready, you might want to discuss feelings of arousal and explain that his body's reactions are completely normal and nothing to feel ashamed of. Talk about ways to handle "spontaneous erections" in public situations. Nocturnal emissions or "wet dreams" are a common occurrence at this age and nothing to be embarrassed about or feel ashamed of.

Puberty is a great time for kids to learn how to use the washer and dryer because they will have sweaty clothes and sheets. Don't forget to mention that frequent (if not daily!) showering will become a must during this time period. Mention that it helps every guy look and feel better. Be positive! Talk about the amazing things the male body can do.

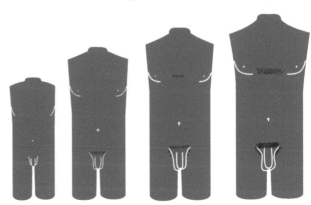

Questions for Your Child

- Have you noticed any changes in your body?
- Are there any changes in your body that you are looking forward to?
- Is there anything about puberty you're confused or nervous about?
- What's the most exciting thing about growing up?
- Have you noticed other kids your age starting to change?
- How would you feel if you didn't start puberty at the same time your friends did?
- Even Jesus Christ had to go through physical and spiritual changes. He "received not of the fulness at first, but continued from grace to grace, until he received a fulness" (D&C 93:12). How do you receive and grow "grace to grace"?

Activity

Talk about Dad's experience with puberty. Discuss his age when he started and how this is some-times an indicator of when a son will begin. Dad, share your experiences.

> "The period of life between four and eleven years comes between two very intense stages of development— early growth and puberty... President David O. McKay said: "The home is the best place in the world to teach the child self-restraint, to give him happiness in self-control, and respect for the rights of others."
>
> –"Home … and the Strength of Youth," (Improvement Era, Aug. 1959, p. 583)

Additional Resources:

"Talking with Your Kids about Puberty: You Got This!" from Educate and Empower Kids
"Talking to our kids about puberty can be awkward! But it doesn't have to be! Tackling tough topics with your kids shows them that they can talk to you about cringy subjects without you freaking out."

"Teaching Children about Physical Development" from the Handbook for Families, June, 1988.
This is a great resource from the Church to help parents discuss physical development, puberty, and more.

"A Foundation for Your Future" from the Liahona, August 2020
"If you want to reach your potential in the future and become the person the Lord wants you to be, you had better keep the eternal big picture in mind and work on it today." –Richard J. Maynes

5. PUBERTY FOR GIRLS

Puberty can be a challenging season as our bodies grow and change so that we can become young women and men. It is the transitional period between childhood and adulthood. Talk openly and positively about these changes that your child is experiencing. Let them know that the changes are normal and that you have gone through them too!

> "But grow in grace, and in the knowledge of our Lord and Saviour Jesus Christ."
>
> —2 Peter 3:18

Discuss the physical changes your daughter can expect: hair growth, increased sweat, breast development, menstruation (see the following lesson). Explain that with newly increased hormones, she is likely to experience some emotional changes. Honestly talk about how feelings of arousal, wetness, and discharge in the vaginal area are normal and natural.

Start the Conversation

Describe how girls begin to grow hair under their arms, in the pubic area, and will experience thicker growth in places like legs and arms. Sweat glands will produce more sweat, and the area under the arms might smell unpleasant. Breasts will become tender and start to develop. Point out that breast development can vary widely in girls and is usually the signal of the onset of puberty. Discuss how emotional and sensitive girls can become during this time due to hormonal changes. If you are discussing this with your daughter and she is ready, you might want to discuss feelings of arousal and explain that her body's reactions are completely normal and nothing to feel ashamed of. Follow up with the next lesson, Menstrual Cycle.

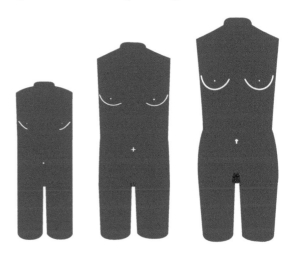

Puberty is a great time to discuss with your daughter the necessity of purchasing bras and picking out deodorant. You may want to teach her how to shave her legs and under arms as well. Don't forget to mention that frequent (if not daily!) showering will become a must during this time period. Remind her that it helps every girl look and feel better. Be sure to talk about the amazing things the female body can do!

Questions for Your Child

- Have you noticed any changes in your body?
- Are there any changes in your body that you are looking forward to?
- Is there anything about puberty you're confused about?
- What changes are you nervous about experiencing?
- If puberty is sometimes uncomfortable or unpleasant, why did God create us in such a way that requires it to happen?
- Growing up can be fun and challenging. How do you picture it?
- Have you talked to any of your friends about these changes? What have you learned?
- What can I do to help you feel more comfortable talking about these changes?

Activity

Mom, tell your daughter about some of your experiences with puberty. If possible, discuss how old you were when you started puberty. Talk about how this is sometimes an indicator of when a daughter will start. Mom, feel free to share the positive and embarrassing parts of your experience.

Additional Resources:

"8 Things Your Daughter Needs to Hear from YOU" from Educate and Empower Kids, Written for mothers to their daughters, this article lists the top eight things that every daughter needs to hear from her mother.

"Helping Your Child Develop Empathy" from Educate and Empower Kids "Empathy is a critical component in developing emotional intelligence. We develop this skill as we become aware of other people's feelings, needs, and concerns. Empathy is important because it helps us to understand how others are feeling and how our actions might impact them."

"Improve Your Relationship with Your Daughter – Here Are Four Ways to Better Communication" from Educate and Empower Kids
This article is to help fathers improve their relationships with their daughters, going over different methods and tips on how to work at that.

6. MENSTRUAL CYCLE

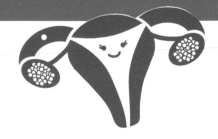 This can be an exciting or terrifying time for a girl. Prepare your daughter by calmly and matter-of-factly discussing the facts. Help her understand the physical effects and emotional shifts that occur during a menstrual cycle. Although many girls don't like having a period, remind your daughter that menstrual cycles make it so women can bear and have children, therefore blessing parents with the joy of having children. If you are discussing this with your son, help him to understand that girls may be sensitive or embarrassed by their periods.

> **Menstrual Period:** *A discharging of blood, secretions, and tissue debris from the uterus as it sheds its thickened lining (endometrium) approximately once per month in females who've reached a fertile age. This does not occur during pregnancy.*

Feel free to share with your daughter when your first menstrual cycle started to help her know it is normal and happens to almost all women. You can also prepare her and have her put feminine products in her backpack in case her period starts unexpectedly.

Start the Conversation

Explain to your child that the age of first menstruation varies widely, with the average age being 12 years old. Point out that discharge (mucus from vagina) may begin about 6 months before the first period.

If you have a diagram, now may be a good time to use it to explain menstruation. First, the egg is released from the ovaries through the fallopian tube into the uterus. Each month, a lining of blood and tissue build up in the uterus. When the egg is not fertilized, this lining is not needed and is shed from the body through the vagina.

A cycle is roughly 28 days but can vary. Bleeding time lasts from 2-7 days. It may be accompanied by cramping, water retention, breast tenderness, and emotional sensitivity. Point out that there is no way of knowing just by looking at a girl if she is menstruating. Being prepared is a young girl's best bet! Talk about the various methods of containing the period to keep clean, such as sanitary napkins or "pads," tampons (with various kinds of applicators and absorbency levels), and menstrual cups, and explain how each is used. Talk about mood changes that can occur around periods, and how each girl reacts differently to these changing hormone levels.

Questions for Your Child

- What have you heard about menstrual periods?
- How do you feel about getting your period?
- How can a girl be prepared for her period?
- How can people show more sensitivity to a girl during her period?
- Most teenage girls do not like having their period. What can you do so that it doesn't feel like a burden?

> *"I am a beloved daughter of Heavenly Parents, with a divine nature and eternal destiny."*
>
> *—Young Women Theme*

Additional Resources:

"Chapter 5: Teaching Adolescents: from Twelve to Eighteen Years" from *A Parent's Guide*
"You should prepare your children for the changes that accompany puberty before these changes actually begin. Puberty is the process by which hormones cause the body to change in ways that make procreation possible. These changes mark the passage from childhood to adulthood. The processes are clean, good, and divinely mandated."

"Great Mother Daughter Relationships–Set a Tone for Awesomeness" from Educate and Empower Kids
This short article offers mothers support and advice for how they can open the door for those uncomfortable conversations with their daughters.

7. PHYSICAL MECHANICS OF SEXUAL INTERCOURSE

Discuss the physical mechanics of sex and any additional information your child may need at this developmental stage. Check the glossary for any definitions you may need such as erection, arousal, clitoris, vaginal secretions, oral sex, anal sex, etc.

Orgasm: *The rhythmic muscular contractions in the pelvic region that occur as a result of sexual stimulation, arousal, and activity during the sexual response cycle. Orgasms are characterized by a sudden release of built-up sexual tension and by the resulting sexual pleasure.*

Allow your child to guide this conversation so you know how much information they are ready for. Make sure your child and you are on the same page by asking your child what they already know about the word "sex" (See Sample Dialogue below). Use your wisdom and experience with this child to gauge how much information they are ready for. If your child seems ready (they mention that kids have been talking about sex on the playground or they ask more specific questions), start with the basics. You may wish to speak in the abstract. "A man and a woman each have body parts that fit together. . ."

Your child will sense if you're uncomfortable, so try to relax! Talk about it matter-of-factly, like you would explain anything to your child!

Start the Conversation

Start off by letting your child know that talking about sex can be uncomfortable or awkward for some people, and it is totally okay to feel awkward. Remind them that you are there to answer their questions, even if they feel awkward.

Describe sexual intercourse. Here are the basics: A man places his erect penis into the vagina of his partner. She may help direct him to make insertion easier. One or both partners may thrust rhythmically until the man or both of them orgasm. When he orgasms, sperm is released from his penis.

Typically, a man helps his partner achieve orgasm before focusing on his orgasm. He helps his partner achieve orgasm by stimulating her genitals, especially her clitoris. As she feels more aroused, her vaginal area will become wet with vaginal secretions. This makes the insertion of the penis easier. With proper stimulation, the woman will orgasm. This can happen before the man places his penis into her vagina.

Let your child know that although simultaneous orgasm is often portrayed in media, often one partner orgasms before the other. Discuss how this might be a better way to have intercourse as it allows one person to focus on the pleasure of their partner and then have their partner focus their attention on them.

Sample Dialogue

Parent: I know that a lot of people feel uncomfortable talking about sex. You may feel uncomfortable and that's a normal response for lots of kids. However, it's really important that you have correct information. I want you to know that you can always come and ask me questions about sex or anything. So, let's make sure we are on the same page. Please tell me what you know about the word sex? (Allow your child to answer.)

Questions for Your Child

- Are your classmates talking about sex? What do you think about this?
- What does the gospel teach us about sexual intimacy? (Discuss respect, kindness, and covenant marriage.)
- Why does God want us to wait until we are married before we have sex?
- What problems and sadness can we avoid by waiting until we are married to have sex?
- God wants us to wait until we are married to have sex, but does this mean sex is bad? (No! It means that there is a right time to start having sex.)

"Sexual feelings are an important part of God's plan to create happy marriages and eternal families. These feelings are not sinful—they are sacred. Because sexual feelings are so sacred and so powerful, God has given you His law of chastity to prepare you to use these feelings as He intends. The law of chastity states that God approves of sexual activity only between a man and a woman who are married. Many in the world ignore or even mock God's law, but the Lord invites us to be His disciples and live a standard higher than the world's."

—For the Strength of Youth: A Guide for Making Choices

Additional Resources:

"8 Ways to Start Talking to Your Child about Sex"
from Educate and Empower Kids
"It can be awkward in the beginning, no doubt, but
discussing sexual intimacy is such an important
conversation that, as parents, we need to use every
healthy way we can to start talking until we find a way
that works."

"Common Mistakes Parents Make When Talking to Kids
about Sex" from Educate and Empower Kids
This article gives some great advice on how to empower
your kids with accurate information.

"How, When, and Why: Talking to Your Children about
Sexuality" from the *Ensign*, August 2020
"To help our children prepare for and enjoy sexuality in
its beauty and wonder within marriage, we need to guide
them as they work toward controlling their God-given
feelings" –Laura M. Padilla-Walker and Meg O. Jankovich

"Teaching about Procreation and Chastity"
from The Family Home Evening Resource Book
We are all children of God with biological parents
and heavenly parents.

"Your Body Is Sacred"
from *For the Strength of Youth: A Guide for Making
Choices*
This section speaks about how to make wise and inspired
choices regarding the sacredness of your own body.

8. EMOTIONAL ASPECTS OF SEX

Through books, movies, social media, and elsewhere, pop culture tends to portray sex as a purely selfish, physical interaction rather than an action based on a strong relationship. Explain that sex can be a natural expression of emotional love, but it can also create feelings of confusion and hurt if not accompanied by love and commitment.

Help your child understand that sexual acts and emotional intimacy can be two separate things, but that God did not intend them to be separated. Sex on its own is usually an empty or selfish experience. Better sexual experiences occur in a committed relationship where both partners have real intimacy, mutual respect, and full confidence in their love. Discuss the amazing, uniting force that sexual intimacy can be in a relationship.

Start the Conversation

Help your child understand the connection between emotions and physical expression such as laughing when we think something is funny, stamping a foot when we feel angry, or wanting a hug when we feel sad. Talk about why we only kiss people we like or love. Remind them of the good feelings we get from hugs. Explain when he or she is ready that these are the same reasons sex is always better in a committed relationship. Reiterate the fact that children are not emotionally ready to have sex. Discuss your family's personal values and beliefs about when and with whom it is appropriate to have sex.

> *"Such an act of love between a man and a woman is—or certainly was ordained to be—a symbol of total union: union of their hearts, their hopes, their lives, their love, their family, their future, their everything."*
>
> *—Jeffrey R. Holland, "Of Souls, Symbols, and Sacraments," 1988.*

Questions for Your Child

- What does "emotional intimacy" feel like? (warmth, happiness, peace, caring, etc.)
- Why does loving someone make people want to express that love in a physical way?
- People often focus on the physical pleasure that sex can bring. What feelings and emotions do you think having sex brings to people?
- Sex often makes us feel bonded and profoundly connected. Why should these feelings be kept sacred until marriage?
- God gave us sex and wants married people to enjoy sexual intimacy together. So why do some people think sex is bad or dirty?

Activity

Read "The Family Proclamation" together, particularly the fourth and fifth paragraphs, and discuss the following statements:

- "We further declare that God has commanded that the sacred powers of procreation are to be employed only between man and woman, lawfully wedded as husband and wife. We declare the means by which mortal life is created to be divinely appointed."

Let your kids know that this means that God has given us sexual intimacy to enjoy and bring us closer together as a married couple.

Additional Resources:

"Today's Family: Protect the Power to Create Life" from "Prophets and Apostles"
"The power of creation—or may we say procreation—is not just an incidental part of the plan... Without it the plan could not proceed. The misuse of it may disrupt the plan... Protect and guard your gift. Your actual happiness is at stake." –Boyd K. Packer

"Intimacy Education Vs Sex Education" from Educate and Empower Kids
This article provides parents with a perspective on how sex education goes beyond the physical aspects of the act and encourages parents to put the topic of sex within the context of relationships and religion as well.

"Your Body Is Sacred" from For the Strength of Youth: A Guide for Making Choices
"Living the law of chastity brings God's approval and personal spiritual power. When you are married, this law will bring greater love, trust, and unity to your marriage."

9. RELATIONSHIPS ARE GOOD AND WONDERFUL

Explain that there are many types of relationships we will experience in our lifetime— friendships, relationships with siblings and parents, romantic relationships, professional relationships, and more. Discuss the enriching, fun, and difficult aspects of various relationships. Talk about the emotional, physical, and spiritual benefits of monogamy.

Start the Conversation

Though there are no perfect indicators of readiness for a romantic relationship, age, maturity level, personal responsibility, and accountability are a good start. Tell your children what you have learned over the years that has helped you determine when someone is ready for a relationship.

> *"Thy friends do stand by thee, and they shall hail thee again with warm hearts and friendly hands."*
>
> *–Doctrine and Covenants 121:9*

Discuss the pervasive trend in our culture to have sex with one or multiple partners throughout life without having any committed relationships. Explain your own opinion along with God's laws on this matter—that sexual relations are meant for people in monogomous, married relationships, which is a relationship between two people and excluding all others. Talk about the emotional benefits (trust, connectedness) and health benefits (less risk of STIs). This is a great time to discuss how relationships are formed and how they progress over time. You may want to share how you met your child's father/mother (see activity below).

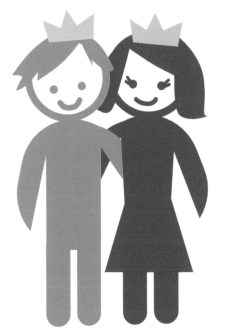

Questions for Your Child

○ What is a relationship?

○ What is the difference between a sibling relationship and a friendship? What is the difference between a friendship and a romantic relationship?

○ Think about your current relationships with your friends and family. Do you treat your family members with the same kindness you treat your friends with?

○ What are some ways we can improve our relationships with our friends? With our siblings? With our parents?

○ As children, you are learning to get along and be a good friend to others. How will this help you in your future relationships? How will this help you to be a good husband or wife?

○ What qualities can a person have that makes being a friend to him or her difficult?

○ How can you get out of a relationship or friendship with someone who is unkind or abusive?

Activity

As a family, talk about the most rewarding relationships you have had with friends, relatives, co-workers, or people at church. Allow each person to talk about a friendship they have really valued. This is a great time to talk about how Mom and Dad met. Allow each person to share at least one experience. What made this relationship fun or special? What makes certain relationships just "click"? What can we do to help relationships grow?

Additional Resources:

Conversations with My Kids: 30 Essential Family Discussions for the Digital Age from Educate and Empower Kids
An amazing resource full of great family night lessons and discussion questions about relationships, LGBTQI issues, compassion, marriage and divorce, lessons on technology, self-improvement, and so much more!

"Make Dating Smooth Sailing" from the *Liahona*, October 2004
"Friendship should play a key role in courtship and marriage. I see friendship as the foundation in the courtship pyramid." –Susan W. Tanner

"Taking the Fear Out of Dating" from the *Ensign*, April 2016
"By understanding and living important principles, you can make your dating experience much more beautiful and successful." –Michael A. Goodman

10. WHAT DOES A HEALTHY RELATIONSHIP LOOK LIKE?

Explain that a healthy relationship includes good communication, mutual respect, kindness, and more. Discuss the healthy aspects of some of your friendships and other relationships. Share why you feel comfortable and loved around certain people and what makes you a good friend or parent.

Use the glossary to discuss physical, emotional, and sexual abuse.

Start the Conversation

Help your child understand that both parties in any relationship are equal. Neither person is above the other and no one, no matter what they have done, deserves to be abused by another person.

Define physical, emotional, and sexual abuse. As you define each of these, allow your child to ask you questions about each of these types of abuse. Share your wisdom and experience. Remind your child that most people are truly good, but that there are bad people in every culture, religion, and neighborhood.

> *"Everyone needs good and true friends. They will be a great strength and blessing to you. They will influence how you think and act, and even help determine the person you will become."*
>
> *—For the Strength of Youth*

Questions for Your Child

- How do healthy relationships begin?
- What are the unique things you could bring to a dating or marriage relationship?
- What qualities do you look for in a friend?
- What qualities might you look for someday in a spouse?
- Someday when you are dating, how will you know you are in a healthy relationship?

- Do you know what abuse looks like?
- What can you do if someone is abusing you? Who can you ask for help?
- What do you think are the differences between a healthy relationship and an abusive one?
- Why is it NOT okay to stay in a relationship where someone hits you even once?
- What adults do you know who have a healthy relationship?
- Why is it important for people in any type of relationship to treat one another with respect?

Sample Dialogue

Parent: Everyone wants and deserves to be loved, and most people want to have a partner that they can share their life with. Someone who they respect and admire, someone they can trust and talk to about anything. What would your ideal person be like? What might they look like? How will you know you have found someone you want to be with forever? (Allow your child to answer.)

Additional Resources:

"Building Meaningful Relationships" from the *Ensign*, August 2018
"The invitation to minister to others is an opportunity to build caring relationships with them . . . When we have made the effort to develop that kind of relationship, God is able to change lives on both sides of the relationship . . . Meaningful relationships aren't tactics. They are built on compassion, sincere efforts, and 'love unfeigned.'"

"How to Create Healthy Relationships" from Educate and Empower Kids
"Teaching children how to build healthy relationships will enable them to recognize when a relationship is unhealthy, build healthy relationships, and allow them to help others to foster healthy relationships."

"Real Life Lessons Learned from Beauty and the Beast" from Educate and Empower Kids
"Many portrayals of boys/men in media allow them a free pass when it comes to their behavior . . . The audience laughs with a 'boys will be boys' attitude. And what about the male character who doesn't take 'no' for an answer, and the audience views it as romantic?"

11. ROMANTIC LOVE

It's essential that our children understand that romantic love is different from physical attraction. Describe how a person can be physically attracted to another without falling in love. Discuss the difference between infatuation and real, long-lasting love.

Make this a fun discussion. Talk about how you fell in love with your spouse and/or about the first time you fell in love. Ask your child to share what they think they might want in a future spouse some day.

Start the Conversation

Tell your child that it is normal to love friends and want to spend time together, but that it's different from romantic love. Give examples of how people express romantic love such as kissing, dating, cuddling, etc. Talk about what romantic love means to you, and discuss that romance is something that happens between people who are older, primarily adults. Ask your child what they think they might feel when they are starting to fall in love.

> Romantic Love: *A form of love that denotes intimacy and a strong desire for emotional connection with another person to whom one is generally also sexually attracted.*

Questions for Your Child

- What do you think romantic love is? How is this different from other kinds of love?
- How do people show romantic love? What do you think falling in love feels like?
- People show love in different ways. How do mom and dad show romantic love?
- What other types of affection have you seen?
- How is love portrayed in TV and movies? Do you think they portray love in a realistic way?
- How do you think a married couple should show love to one another?
- Why do you think the Church recommends that kids should wait until they are 16 to begin dating?
- How will you know you're ready to be in a romantic relationship?

Activity

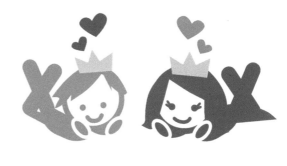

Watch a family-friendly love story such as *The Sound of Music*, *Sense and Sensibility*, *The Princess Bride*, *Ever After*, *Anne of Avonlea*, or one of your favorites. Throughout the movie or afterward, ask your child the following questions:

- Do these characters seem like anyone we know in real life?
- Is this a realistic depiction of how people fall in love?
- Is this how you would like to fall in love?
- Do you think their relationship will last?
- How do you think you will know you are in love with someone?

Additional Resources:

"The Gospel and Romantic Love" from the *New Era*, February 2002
"The scriptures counsel us to be virtuous not because romantic love is bad, but precisely because romantic love is so good. It is not only good; it is pure, precious, even sacred and holy. For that reason, one of Satan's cheapest and dirtiest tricks is to make profane that which is sacred." –Bruce C. Hafen

"A Wedding Dress and a Plan" from the *Liahona*, April 2010
This is the story of a girl learning about the significance of her older sister's temple wedding.

"Beyond the Sex Talk: Teaching Teens Emotional Intimacy" from Educate and Empower Kids
Working well as a follow-up for our article, "Intimacy Education Vs Sex Education," this article offers parents several ways to discuss with their teens the role that emotional intimacy plays in physical intimacy.

"Teaching Children: from Four to Eleven Years" from *A Parent's Guide*
"To a large extent the child feels these emotions naturally. . . . You and your spouse can be your children's best examples of intimate relationships."

> *"Thou shalt love thy wife with all thy heart, and shalt cleave unto her and none else."*
>
> *–Doctrine and Covenants 42:22*

"What Is the Law of Chastity?" from the *New Era*, August 2019
"Note that the Lord's standards don't change just because two people really like each other and both agree to the behavior. When you respect other people, the Lord, and yourself, you'll keep the commandments." –Joshua J. Perkey

12. DIFFERENT KINDS OF FAMILIES

There are many different kinds of families. Some kids are raised by grandparents, aunts and uncles, or other family members. Some children are raised by a single parent. Some families have two dads or two moms, and some kids are raised by one mother and one father. Discuss some of the families you know that are different from yours.

This may be a great time to look at your family's history on familysearch. org. Show your kids the variety of families they have come from. Feel free to talk about some of the different traditions and behaviors you can decipher from studying family history (like people marrying their cousins, staying in one town for generations, naming their children in a certain way, etc.).

> *"Pray in your families unto the Father, always in my name, that your wives and your children may be blessed."*
>
> *–3 Nephi 18:21*

Start the Conversation

Every family is different and special in its own way. It is important that we love our friends and those we interact with regardless of their family circumstances. Talk with your child about how important family is, and that we should never put down friends for having a different family than ours. There

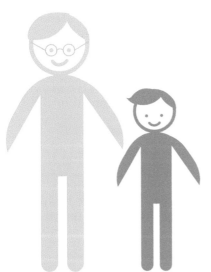

is no such thing as a perfect family. Discuss the different kinds of families you see at church, school, and in your neighborhood. Make sure to emphasize that everyone has gifts and challenges, and that every family is unique and special. Although families come in different shapes and sizes, they all have value and each family member is a child of God, just like you and your child.

Discuss "The Family: A Proclamation to the World." Talk about the best situation for raising children–with two parents–but that God accepts, loves, and helps EVERY family no matter their circumstances. Read the paragraph where it says, "we warn that the disintegration of the family will bring upon individuals, communities, and nations the calamities foretold by ancient and modern prophets." Ask your child what the "disintegration of the family" means. What can we do to prevent this?

Questions for Your Child

Q How could you describe your family?

Q Tell me what you imagine your future family will be like? How will that family be similar to your family now? How will it be different?

Q What makes a strong family? What can we do to make our family stronger?

Q Why does God command us to honor our parents?

Q How does doing this strengthen our family?

Q Whether you are being raised by your grandparents, two parents, or one, why does God care so much about families? Why do our heavenly parents want our families to be eternal?

Activity

Read or Sing "The Family Is of God." Ask your children why mothers and fathers each have special importance in raising children. Explain why families are the most important unit in the Church and in society.

Additional Resources:

"And as I partook of the fruit thereof it filled my soul with exceedingly great joy; wherefore, I began to be desirous that my family should partake of it also; for I knew that it was desirable above all other fruit." –1 Nephi 8:12

"Different Kinds of Families" from the *Ensign*, July 2018

"Families are part of Heavenly Father's plan. Like people, they come in different shapes and sizes. Sometimes it may seem like there are 'perfect families' all around us, but in reality, this world is made up of imperfect people in family units just trying to figure things out . . . [N]o family is perfect!"

"The Family" from the *Liahona*, October 1998

"We begin to practice in the family, the smaller unit, what will spread to the Church and to the society in which we live in this world, which will then be what we practice in families bound together forever by covenants and by faithfulness." –Henry B. Eyring

13. GENDER & GENDER ROLES

Throughout history, gender roles have evolved in many different ways. As our culture explores what it means to be a woman and what it means to be a man, it's important to teach our kids how we can elevate the status of women and girls without devaluing men and boys. Teach your kids how in their grandparents' youth, girls had much fewer educational opportunities and were expected to take on most of the responsibility of raising children. Nowadays, parents share the responsibilities of raising children and running a household.

At church, at school, at work, and in our families, we sometimes let stereotypical gender roles stop us from trying something new or speaking up on certain topics. Discuss the division of indoor and outdoor chores for your home and your thoughts of the various roles and responsibilities of men and women. Talk about the strengths of various men and women you know.

Start the Conversation

Encourage a good conversation about stereotyping and typical male and female roles. Remind your kids that although our bodies and physical abilities are different in fundamental ways, women and men can perform mental, emotional, and spiritual tasks equally well. Share your personal thoughts.

Gender Role: *The pattern of masculine or feminine behavior of an individual that is defined by a particular culture and that is largely determined by a child's upbringing.*

Ask: How do both of your parents contribute to your home and family? Both boys and girls are necessary in our families, wards, and communities. What are some ways you would like to contribute to your family and community?

Explain to your kids that the world's ideas about gender, gender expression, and gender identity are changing rapidly! But the Lord's truths about gender, as outlined in "The Family Proclamation" still hold true: "Gender is an essential characteristic of individual premortal, mortal, and eternal identity and purpose." Explain to your child that of all their various identities (Christian, American, Asian, male, female, etc), their most important identity is that of a child of heavenly parents.

Questions for Your Child

Q Are there typical boy and girl interests?

Q Is it okay for boys and girls to pursue whatever activities they are interested in doing?

Q Is it okay for boys to be interested in what are thought of as feminine things and for girls to be interested in typically masculine things?

Q Why is it important to look past a friend's likes or outward appearance, and instead focus on who they really are?

Q Before you came to Earth, you were a boy or a girl. What makes a girl a girl? What makes a boy a boy?

Q Boy or girl, you are a child of heavenly parents. How will knowing your eternal identity bless your life?

> *"And the Gods took counsel among themselves and said: Let us go down and form man in our image, after our likeness . . . So the Gods went down to organize man in their own image, in the image of the Gods to form they him, male and female to form they them."*
>
> *—Abraham 4:26-27*

Additional Resources:

"That by him, and through him, and of him, the worlds are and were created, and the inhabitants thereof are begotten sons and daughters unto God." –D&C 76:24

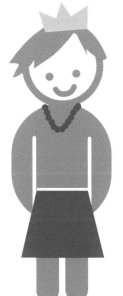

"How the fetus actually becomes male or female is important information for parents and children. Soon after conception, all children have internal and external sex organs in a simple form . . . This differentiation between the two genders–male and female–progresses throughout physiological development until there are complete internal and external female or male reproductive organs. The reproductive organs that develop while in the womb for the male fetus include testes . . . the penis . . . and the scrotum. . . . The female fetus develops two ovaries (which contain all the egg cells she will have during a lifetime); the uterus (womb) . . .; the vagina . . .;and labia. . . . At birth the male or the female infant has reproductive organs but lacks reproductive capacity. This comes at puberty." –A Parents Guide

"The Family: A Proclamation to the World"

"In these sacred responsibilities, fathers and mothers are obligated to help one another as equal partners."

"Teaching Children: from Four to Eleven Years" from A Parent's Guide

"By teaching your children these eternal roles, you help them organize their thoughts and behavior around a nucleus of righteous values. These values naturally place sexual interests and information in an eternal perspective."

14. SEXUAL IDENTIFICATION

This is a great opportunity to teach your kids about the various kinds of sexual identifications. Your child has probably already heard something of one or more of them. Define each one and be ready to answer your child's questions.

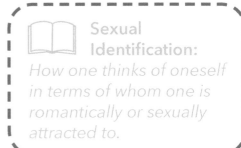

Sexual Identification: How one thinks of oneself in terms of whom one is romantically or sexually attracted to.

Use the glossary to help you discuss heterosexual, gay, lesbian, bisexual, transgender, asexual, and intersex identifications.

Start the Conversation

First, explain the difference between friend love and sexual attraction. Make it clear that liking someone or being a fan of someone who is gay (a friend or on TV) does not make someone gay. You can even love your friends without being "in love" with them.

With so much hypersexualized media and pornography available to kids, media can sometimes influence how a child or teen sees themselves sexually. Sometimes a friend's sexual identity or pressuring parents can influence one's sexual identity. Teach your child that no one's sexuality should be influenced by anyone or anything else. Ask your child what his or her thoughts are on the subject.

Describe how identifying oneself as any particular sexuality does not strictly define a person. One's sexuality is an integral part of them, but it does not define who they are. Remind your child that of all their identities (boy, girl, Latter-day Saint, gay, straight, Latino, etc.), their most important identity is that of being a child of God. Explain that as your child faces hardships, life questions, or criticisms from others, it is always helpful to remember that they and everyone around them are children of God. Ask your child how knowing they are a child of God can be helpful when one is feeling sad or overwhelmed.

Note: Reiterate that we should never mistreat people for being different or having a different sexual identity as you! Share your personal thoughts and understanding of the topic.

Questions for Your Child

- How do you like to be treated? How do you treat those who are gay, lesbian, or straight?
- What do your classmates and teachers say about homosexuality?
- What should you do if you experience feelings of same sex attraction? Who is a trusted loved one that you can talk to about this?
- What does LGBTQI stand for?
- What does it mean to be gay?
- How are gay people and straight people different?
- How are those who identify as gay (or any of the other terms listed above) not different from others at all?

> *"A new commandment I give unto you, That ye love one another; as I have loved you . . .*
> *By this shall all men know that ye are my disciples, if ye have love one to another."*
>
> *–John 13:34-35*

Additional Resources:

"Starting Conversations with Your Kids about LGBTQ Identities" from Educate and Empower Kids

"It is important to teach through behavior and conversation that treating others with respect is critical to our communities. This will lead to more tolerance and safety for all people no matter their identity."

"What do I need to understand about same-sex attraction?" from the *Same-Sex Attraction Manual*

"Attraction is not identity. People can make their own choices about how to identify. . . .There are active Church members who experience same-sex attraction and never choose to identify themselves using a label. Our primary identity will always be as a child of God."

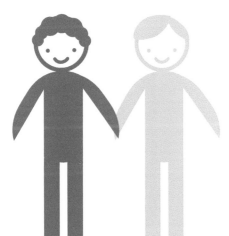

"The Lord's Plan for Men and Women" from the *Ensign*, October 1975

"The bodies of men and the bodies of women were created differently so they complemented each other, so that the union of the two would bring a conception which would bring a living soul into the world."
–Spencer W. Kimball

"We Are More Than Our Labels" from *YA Weekly*, August 2018

"While labels empower us, boost our sense of identity, and allow us opportunities for growth, there is also a dangerous side to them" –Chakell Wardleigh, Chaleese Leishman, and Chantele Sedgwick

15. AT WHAT AGE IS SOMEONE READY FOR A SEXUAL RELATIONSHIP?

> *"Let virtue garnish thy thoughts unceasingly; then shall thy confidence wax strong in the presence of God"*
>
> *–Doctrine and Covenants 121:45*

Discuss with your child the various stages of a physical relationship: hand-holding, hugging, kissing, petting, sexual intercourse. Explain that people are ready for these stages at different ages, but that there are reasons why the *For the Strength of Youth* encourages dating after the age of 16. Talk about these reasons. Point out that teenagers are not emotionally ready for sexual relationships, and that children are neither physically nor emotionally ready either.

Remind your children that God gave us sexual intimacy, curiosity, and sexual desires. These are natural, good things. Sex is beautiful and good, but it is to be saved for marriage.

Start the Conversation

Teach the natural physical progression of a HEALTHY sexual relationship. Explain that a healthy sexual relationship is one in which both parties feel equally respected. Talk about how most healthy marriages start off as friendships and begin with smaller acts of intimacy (kissing, hugging, cuddling) before moving on to more intimate acts like sexual intercourse.

Discuss the aspects that show one is ready for dating, marriage, and sex. These may include: age, maturity level, capabilities, and personal responsibility. Reiterate your personal or family standards on this subject.

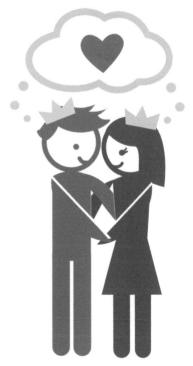

Questions for Your Child

- What factors should be considered to determine if someone is ready for sex?

- Many teenagers are having sex at younger and younger ages. Why do you think that is?

- At what age do you think it is okay to start having sex? Is there a right age for everyone?

- What are the benefits of waiting to have sex until you are married?

- What personal habits and rules can you make for yourself to make sure you remain sexually pure until marriage?

- How can learning to listen to the Holy Ghost help you stay sexually pure?

- Someday you will be dating. What can you do if someone is pressuring you to have sex and you do not want to?

Additional Resources:

"[B]ridle all your passions, that ye may be filled with love." –Alma 38:12

"Personal Purity" from the *Ensign*, November 1998

"[H]uman intimacy is reserved for a married couple because it is the ultimate symbol of total union, a totality and a union ordained and defined by God . . . marriage was intended to mean the complete merger of a man and a woman–their hearts, hopes, lives, love, family, future, everything . . . This is a union of such completeness that we use the word seal to convey its eternal promise." –Jeffrey R. Holland

"Talking to Your Parents about Sex" from the *New Era*, August 2020

"At first it might be awkward to talk with your parents or another trusted adult. Remember, your Heavenly Father loves you and wants you to prepare to develop a healthy relationship as an adult. Part of your preparation includes understanding healthy, appropriate sexuality and learning how to communicate about it now." –Derek Willis Hagey

"Sexual Purity" from *For the Strength of Youth*

"The Lord's standard regarding sexual purity is clear and unchanging. Do not have any sexual relations before marriage, and be completely faithful to your spouse after marriage."

"Yes, You Can: The True Power of Sexual Purity" from the *New Era*, June 2017

"When it comes to sexual purity, you might think that the world is full of cans, and the gospel is full of can'ts. But it's just the opposite." –By Charlotte Larcabal

16. CURIOSITY

Teach your child that curiosity about sex, your developing body, and other's bodies is normal and God-given. Your children are going to have questions about sex. Being a good source for them to come to and ask those questions is essential for their understanding and decision making.

Emphasize to your kids that they should never feel ashamed for being curious, and let them know they can talk to you anytime they feel curious about anything they might have questions about. Explain why parents are

> "Fear not; ask questions. Be curious, but doubt not! Always hold fast to faith and to the light you have already received."
>
> –Dieter F. Uctdorf

the best source of information and how friends at school often have wrong or only partially correct information. You will find more helpful information regarding curiosity when you teach lesson #23, "Pornography."

Start the Conversation

It's so important that children never be made to feel embarrassed for being curious. It's completely natural! Validate your child's awareness and answer questions honestly and completely. Make them feel as comfortable as possible when they come to you with questions. Remind them that your home is a safe zone where questions are always okay. If some topics are too awkward to ask questions about face to face, give your kids the option to write it down.

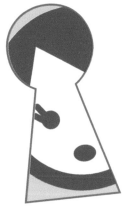

Questions for Your Child

Q Why is curiosity a good thing?

Q Who should you talk to if you are curious about your body? About sex? About members of the opposite gender?

Q How is curiosity essential to learning?

Q How is curiosity essential to gaining a testimony of the gospel of Jesus Christ?

Q What are some things about your body that you are curious about?

Q What else are you curious about?

Q Would you like to know more about (pick your own topic) ?

Q What can I do to help you feel more comfortable coming to me with questions?

Activity

Share an experience with your child about a time you were curious about something.

Q How did you find more information?

Q Was this a good experience or not?

Q Did your parents have any particular reaction to your curiosity?

Q Were you able to ask your parents awkward questions?

Additional Resources:

"Teaching Without Shame: Understanding Your Child's Curiosity" from Educate and Empower Kids

This article tells the story of a mother talking through her son's curiosity with him and helping him understand that our bodies are beautiful and natural, but that we each deserve our own privacy as well.

"How to Teach Children about Sexual Intimacy" from *Church News*

"If we understand healthy sexuality in the context of it being divine, we are tying into our divine identity and our divine potential and the divine potential of our spouse and of our eternal family." –Lee Gibbons

"God's Power Within You", from the *Friend*, January 2002

President Gordon B. Hinckley talks about facing and overcoming temptations.

17. MASTURBATION

There are many opinions about masturbation in the world. Some doctors and researchers say it is a healthy activity for kids and adults and that it is a normal part of a child's development. However the Church teaches the Lord's standard which says that masturbation is a self-interested and unnecessary behavior. If you believe that masturbation is unhealthy or spiritually harmful, tell your child and explain WHY. Reading the section Sexual Purity in the *For the Strength of Youth* pamphlet may be helpful.

Since masturbation often accompanies pornography viewing, you may wish to discuss this lesson in conjunction with lesson #23, Pornography. Please also keep in mind that many young children explore their genitals or masturbate for the simple reason that it feels good. They may not even be trying to achieve orgasm. This discussion is different and for an older child that understands the "purpose" of masturbation.

> *"When you are sexually pure, you prepare yourself to make and keep sacred covenants in the temple."*
>
> *—For the Strength of Youth*

Start the Conversation

Explain that masturbation is self-stimulation of the genitals and that most people do it to achieve orgasm. Discuss your personal views with your child about masturbation. Explain that it can be a habit-forming behavior. Talk about the impulses kids start feeling around puberty and how normal and natural those feelings are. Talk about healthy ways they can handle those impulses.

However you choose to talk about masturbation with your child, it is important to avoid shaming your child. Let them know that they are loved. Remember, some kids are simply using masturbation to explore their bodies or to relax. Explain that although it is considered a sinful behavior, a person who masturbates is NOT bad or evil. Remind your child that if they engage in any sinful behavior, you will still love them!

Questions for Your Child

○ Do you understand what masturbation is?

○ Is it healthy to explore our bodies? What is the difference between masturbating and exploring?

○ Is masturbation good? Bad? Neither? If you masturbate, are you a bad person? (No!)

○ What other activities could you do if you are tempted to masturbate (read a book, go on a walk, play a game, talk to a friend, draw, bake, etc.)?

○ Are there consequences if masturbation becomes a habit?

○ Who can you talk to if this becomes a habit in your life?

○ Many people often feel ashamed of masturbating, so they hide what they are doing. How does hiding a habit make it more difficult to overcome?

Additional Resources:

"Talking to Your Children about Moral Purity" from the *Ensign*, December 1986
"Children should be taught, at around the first signs of puberty, what masturbation is and why it is wrong. Parents who avoid guiding their children in this matter do them a disservice. Masturbation can be described as manipulating one's own sexual organs to produce sexual excitement. Such practice 'is not approved of the Lord nor of his church.'" –Spencer W. Kimball

"Talking with Our Kids about Masturbation—Without Shame!" from Educate and Empower Kids

This article offers parents a variety of ways that they can choose to approach discussing masturbation.

"Talking with Our Daughters about Masturbation" from Educate and Empower Kids

This article discusses how parents can approach their daughters specifically about the topic of masturbation.

"Masturbation and Kids–Moving Beyond the Shame!" from Educate and Empower Kids

This article tells of the impacts masturbation can have on one's childhood and adulthood. This author also provides parents with suggestions on how they can teach their own children about masturbation without guilt or shame.

"Overcoming Your Challenges" from the *Friend*, March 2022

"I promise that Heavenly Father will help you overcome your challenges. He loves you and will help you become what He wants you to become." –President Dallin H. Oaks

18. CHILDREN DO NOT HAVE SEX

It may seem like common sense that children do not have sex. However, as kids are exposed to pornography and hypersexualized media, and they spend large amounts of time online, something as basic as this needs to be taught!

> When His disciples asked, "Who is the greatest in the kingdom of heaven? ... Jesus called a little child unto him, and set him in the midst of them, and said, ... Whosoever ... shall humble himself as this little child, the same is greatest in the kingdom of heaven."
>
> –Matthew 18:1–5

As a family, create a plan of what your kids can do if someone touches them inappropriately, tries to show them pornography, tries to be alone with them, or any other situation that you think your children should be prepared for. This and the following lessons have several teaching points to guide you.

Start the Conversation

Explain to your child that an adult you can trust will never say it is normal for a child to have sex. Children's bodies are not physically mature or ready for sex. Children also have a different emotional capability than adults. These are reasons why children DO NOT have sex. Share these reasons with your child. Remind your child that sex is for grown-ups. Not kids. It is against the law for someone to have sex with a child. Teach your kids you ALWAYS have the right to say, "NO!"

Questions for Your Child

Q Has anyone ever touched you in a place that is covered by your bathing suit?

Q Has anyone told you to take off your clothes except for mom and dad?

Q What can you do if someone tries to touch you in a place that is covered by your bathing suit?

- Ninety percent of sexual abuse is perpetrated by people we know (a friend, step-sibling, a coach, uncle, etc.). Who are the few people that we trust with absolute certainty? (This should be a very small list of 2-5 people that your kids can rely on with 100% confidence.)

- What should you do if someone tells you that sex is normal for children? Why do you think someone would say that?

- What should you do if someone asks you to have sex or tries to touch the private parts of your body? Has this ever happened to you?

- What should you do if a friend tells you they are being sexually abused by someone? Who can you talk to?

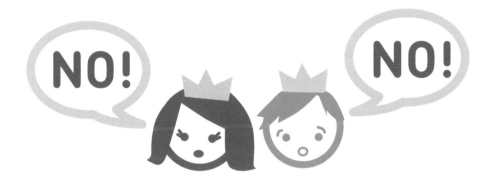

Additional Resources:

"Youth Speak Out on Sexual Purity" from the *New Era*, April 2016

A series of testimonials from youth on the importance of sexual purity.

"My Body is Mine: Teaching Kids Appropriate Touch" from Educate and Empower Kids

"Teaching your children about appropriate touch will empower them to stand up for themselves and their bodies."

"Teaching Consent. Starting Early and Simply." from Educate and Empower Kids

"[W]e can start teaching our children about consent at a young age by teaching respect for others and boundaries, which are all vital components of a child's developing healthy sexuality."

"Three Generations of Silence: How Do We Turn This Around?" from Educate and Empower Kids

This article discusses how sexual assault/harassment is something that is often brushed under the rug. It offers a variety of ways that mothers can help ensure that their daughters know when to speak up.

19. WHAT TO DO IF SOMETHING HAS HAPPENED TO YOU: WHO TO TALK TO

Teach your child that if something happens to them that makes them feel uncomfortable or hurts them, they can ALWAYS tell you, that you are on their side, and that you love them no matter what. Be specific in defining what it means to feel uncomfortable –feeling or causing discomfort or unease; disquieting. Give your child examples of times you felt uncomfortable or bring up a time you observed that your child was uncomfortable.

Remind your child that they should always tell someone right away if they are ever touched in a way that makes him or her feel uncomfort-

> "To sexually abuse someone is a serious and grievous sin. If you have been a victim of sexual abuse in any form, at any age, under any circumstances, know that the abuse is not your fault. Heavenly Father and Jesus Christ weep with you. They desperately want to help you find peace and healing."
>
> –Gospel Living

able. Discuss who some trustworthy adults are in your family's life. These can include doctors, police officers, and parents. However, teach your child that no one should make anyone feel uncomfortable, not even trusted adults.

Start the Conversation

Make sure your child understands that if they report that someone has touched them inappropriately, they are NOT in trouble. Explain why it is important to tell a trusted adult. It's important to look for physical cues here. Inform your child that it's important to tell right away, but also that it's never too late. Give reassurance that he or she will be believed. Talk about the adults in your child's life who you trust. Ask your child to list a few people who they trust. Confirm or correct the people on this list. Remind your child that sometimes kids touch or abuse other kids. Discuss with your child what can be done in these circumstances.

Questions for Your Child

- ❑ Other than getting a spanking from a parent, have you ever been hurt by a grown up or older child before? ("Hurt" can mean hitting, slapping, screaming, calling someone terrible names, touching someone on their private parts, etc.)

- ❑ Has any adult ever told you not to tell Mom or Dad something?

- ❑ Why is it a poor choice to keep secrets from your parents?

- ❑ Has anyone ever touched you, talked to you, or shown you something sexual that made you feel uncomfortable?

- ❑ What would you do if this happened to you?

- ❑ Who are adults we can trust? Is there anyone who makes you uncomfortable?

Activity

Talk about what to do if your child reports inappropriate behavior to an adult, only to have it be brushed aside. Discuss options in this scenario like finding another adult or calling someone on their trusted adults list.

Additional Resources:

"Sexual abuse of children is one of the ugliest and personally devastating experiences a child may have . . . When child abuse, including incest, is discovered, care must be taken to know and observe the laws of the Church and of the state in such matters. Priesthood leaders and LDS Social Services workers can be consulted in such cases.

"Parents are not to abuse their children in any way—physically, emotionally, or sexually. Parents who deal with each other in kindness and in a thoughtful manner will create an attitude toward their children of loving concern and patience. Parents and children should learn that normal relationships consist of kindly words and caresses and that firm yet reasonable discipline generally will prevent child abuse. One of the surest preven-tives against child abuse is for the family to know how to speak to and touch each other affectionately without harmful or sexual meaning." *—A Parents Guide*

"Helping Your Child Become the Master of Their Body: Moving beyond Good Touch/ Bad Touch" from Educate and Empower Kids

This family night lesson will guide you in how to help your kids feel comfortable and in control of their bodies, danger signs to look for from predators, how to help your child say "no" to unwanted affection, and more.

"Vigilant Parenting in the Digital Age" from Educate and Empower Kids

"Simply telling our children how to act on the internet is just not enough. We need to be aware of the dangers around, as well as be vigilant in monitoring technology use in our homes . . . We also must have many discussions with our children about technology use, including dangers, safety, and digital citizenship."

20. HOW PREDATORS GROOM CHILDREN

This can be a tough lesson to discuss with your kids, but it may be one of the most important lessons you ever teach. We highly recommend reading our short article "8 Ways a Predator Might Groom Your Child" as you prepare.

Groom: *To prepare or train someone for a particular purpose or activity. In the case of sexual predators, it is any willful action made by the offender to prepare the victim and/ or the victim's support network that allows for easier sex offending.*

Help your child understand what it means for someone to groom a child or teenager. Be real and honest! Discuss common grooming techniques with your child. Define what it means to be a predator—a sexual predator is someone who seeks to obtain sexual contact through pursuing, grooming, and/or hunting.

Be frank with your child. Let them know that predators are often people the child knows. Teach them what it means to listen to your instincts. Remind your children that they should never keep secrets about sex from parents.

Start the Conversation

Explain to your kids that predators may seek to gain the victim's trust, then start to desensitize the child to physical touch by using innocent, affectionate touch, such as a pat on the back or a squeeze of an arm. Predators can sometimes be "friends" or peers. They will seek to isolate their victims and/ or seek to fill a void in the child's life. Remind your child that no one has a right to touch him or her without his or her consent, not even relatives or grown-up friends.

Talk specifically about your family's policies for taking rides, texting, private messaging, and spending time alone with adults and teens who are not on the "trusted adults list." This is also a good time to talk about online predators who might contact your kids through gaming sites, social media, etc. Emphasize the need to be honest with you about their online behavior and to never speak to strangers online—even if they seem to be other kids.

Finally, you must teach your child that if a peer or adult hurts or abuses them, it is not your child's fault. It is the fault of the perpetrator.

Questions for Your Child

- Q Do predators look a certain way? Are they always adults? Do they look ugly and mean, or do they look like everyone else?

- Q When a predator is trying to get you to do something, how might he or she act? Kind? Charming? Friendly?

- Q Is it possible for a predator to be at church? At school?

- Q It's rare for a stranger to try to take a child from a park, mall, or elsewhere. But why should we never get into cars or go anywhere with strangers?

- Q What are some warning signs we can look for in adults or teens? (progressive inappropriate touch, privately texting your child, etc.)

- Q What are some ways we can stay safe from online predators?

"You may feel threatened by one who is in a position of power or control over you. You may feel trapped and see no escape. Please believe that your Heavenly Father does not want you to be held captive by unrighteous influence, by threats of reprisal, or by fear of repercussion to the family member who abuses you. Trust that the Lord will lead you to a solution."

–Richard G Scott, "Healing the Tragic Scars of Abuse," General Conference, April 1992

Activity

Read and discuss Genesis 39, the story of Joseph fleeing Potipher's wife. Talk about her attempts to groom him in verses 7, and 10-12. Discuss his bravery in fleeing from her.

Additional Resources:

"A Lesson for Teaching Your Children about Predators" from Educate and Empower Kids
A simple family night lesson to help parents teach their children about predators.

"What Online Predators Don't Want YOU to Do" from Educate and Empower Kids
This article provides a few tips on what you can do to prevent a predator's access to your kids.

"Abuse: Help, Healing, and Protection"
This page is a portal to many resources and options dedicated to helping victims of abuse.

21. HOW TO SAY "NO"

Saying "no" to an adult can be very difficult for a child. How often were you comfortable saying "no" to an adult when you were a child? Thus, it is essential that you practice and give your kids scenarios where it is okay, and even smart, to say "no."

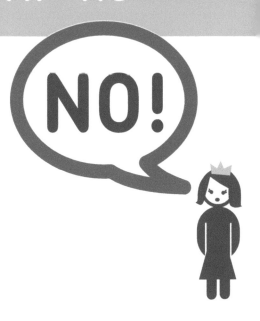

Explain when you expect your children to be obedient—for example, when asked to clean a room or do the dishes. But make it clear to them that there are times when they'll need to have the courage to say "NO!" to an adult.

Sometimes a child may engage in something inappropriate without realizing its repercussions. They may play a game of "show me yours and I'll show you mine" not fully realizing until later that this is a poor choice. Explain that even if they have done something in the past, it doesn't mean they have to do it again.

> *"Have not I commanded thee? Be strong and of a good courage; be not afraid, neither be thou dismayed: for the Lord thy God is with thee whithersoever thou goest."*
>
> *–Joshua 1:9*

Start the Conversation

Discuss different types of dangerous situations your child may encounter, such as when he or she is made to feel uncomfortable by what someone does or says. Talk about which situations your child can say "no" in, not just who they can say "no" to. Teach your child that they have the power to say "no" to anyone. Practice saying "no" loudly and firmly. Then practice yelling "NO!"

43

Questions for Your Child

- Saying "no" to a grown up like a coach or a friend's parent can be very difficult. What can we do to be brave enough to do this?

- What are some instances where we should say "no"? (When someone tries to share drugs or alcohol with us, tries to show us pornography, when an adult tries to get us to be alone with them, when an older child tries to touch us inappropriately, etc.)

- Have you ever had to tell a friend, loved one, or an adult "no"?

- What can you say or do if someone tries to touch you on the private areas of your body, tries to take your clothes off, or tries to take your picture when you are wearing a bathing suit or less clothes? (Yell NO! and run to a safe adult.)

- What are some other circumstances where you can say "no"?

Activity

Create a plan with your child. Ask them what they can do if they are at a friend's house and an older kid or adult makes them feel uncomfortable, tries to get them alone, etc.

- Can they call you and say a "safe word" that your family has agreed on? What else can your child do?

Additional Resources:

"Kids and "Affection": Why I'm NOT Teaching My Kids to Be Polite" from Educate and Empower Kids

This article outlines the importance of helping kids say "no" to unwanted affection and letting them know that they will be believed if something does happen.

"Protecting Children" from the *Ensign*, April 2019

"You could help your children practice saying, 'No!' when someone tries to convince them to do something that makes them uncomfortable. Every child should know that they can ask for help, and they should keep asking until they are safe." –Marissa Widdison

"How to Say No" from the *Friend*, August 2021

This is a practice lesson teaching kids how to say "no" when asked to break the Word of Wisdom.

"Can You Spot the Grooming Behaviors of a Predator?" from Educate and Empower Kids

This lesson teaches a few tactics on how to recognize grooming behaviors and has multiple links to more helpful resources.

22. YOUR INSTINCTS AND THE HOLY GHOST KEEP YOU SAFE

Teach your child that he or she has instincts to help them, along with the gift of the Holy Ghost to guide them. Instincts are a part of us and can keep us safe and can help us make good decisions.

Our book, _This Is the Spirit of Revelation_, is a great resource to help your kids hear, understand, and act upon the promptings of the Holy Ghost.

Parents, it is crucial that you remind your kids of some of the teachings in the lesson How Predators Groom Children (lesson #20). You must explain that even if the Holy Ghost or one's instincts (gut feelings) prompt them to get out of a situation and they don't, if an adult or peer hurts or abuses them in any way, it is still NOT your child's fault. It is the fault of the perpetrator.

Start the Conversation

To describe instincts, bring up a scenario for your child like seeing a big spider or snake or someone jumping out to scare you. Ask your child if he or she has ever had "gut" or instinctual feelings, either positive or negative. This may feel like an "icky" feeling. Ask your child what that "icky" feeling is trying to tell them. Talk about how we can be more sensitive to these feelings.

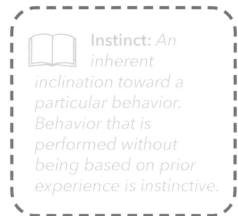

Instinct: _An inherent inclination toward a particular behavior. Behavior that is performed without being based on prior experience is instinctive._

Instincts are similar to an alarm system that we can feel in a dangerous or uncomfortable situation. Teach your child that it is very important that they trust their instincts. Explain that they cannot ignore them just because they don't want to make the person feel bad. Their safety is more important!

Discuss the power of the Holy Ghost. Explain that the Holy Ghost can give us mild, quiet impressions or loud, urgent impressions. These impression may be words you feel rather than hear.

Sometimes we feel prompted to say something or take action. A prompting can be a strong feeling, a warm feeling, or even a peaceful feeling. The Holy Ghost can also be a Comforter, can reveal truth to us, and can protect us by warning us. Remember, sometimes we might hear a voice inside us, but more likely, it will be a voice we feel.

"Verily I say unto you, I will impart unto you of my Spirit, which shall enlighten your mind, which shall fill your soul with joy."

–Doctrine and Covenants 11:13

Questions for Your Child

- ○ What do instincts feel like?
- ○ What are some times or places that our instincts may try to warn us?
- ○ How have you felt the Holy Ghost in your life?
- ○ What are some of the ways the Holy Ghost speaks to people?
- ○ How can you increase the Holy Ghost's presence in your life?

Activity

Mom or Dad, share a story from your life about when the Spirit prompted you to do something. Did you listen or not? What was the consequence of that action?

Additional Resources:

"And it came to pass when they heard this voice, and beheld that it was not a voice of thunder, neither was it a voice of a great tumultuous noise, but behold, it was a still voice of perfect mildness, as if it had been a whisper, and it did pierce even to the very soul." –Helaman 5:30

"Let the Holy Spirit Guide" from general conference, April 2017

"To give us mortal strength and divine guidance, [our Father in Heaven] provided the Holy Spirit." –Ronald A. Rasband

"Obeying the Whisperings of the Holy Ghost" from the *Ensign*, August 2007

"The blessings, insights, and protection we receive when we are obedient are beyond our comprehension . . . [T]he Spirit can help us avoid temptation and ultimately spiritual death if we listen and respond." –Ronald T. Halverson

Chloe Has a Question. A Very Important Question by Dina Alexander

A fun story and workbook! With her family's help, Chloe learns one of the most important lessons in gospel living: Questions aren't just good, they are great!

"The Secret I Almost Did Not Tell" from Educate and Empower Kids

In this article, the author talks about her own experience with sexual assault as a child and what parents can do to help stop it.

23. PORNOGRAPHY

Pornography (porn) is where our children and teens are learning some of the most repugnant, unhealthy messages about sex, love, relationships, and body image. It is damaging to individuals, relationships, and society. This is such an important lesson! Please take plenty of time to discuss this lesson, and don't be afraid to repeat it.

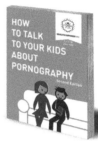

Develop a plan for what to do if your child is exposed to pornography. Use our RUN Plan Family Night Lesson, found at educateempowerkids.org, to create a plan for the next time your child is exposed to pornography.

For more detailed help, check out our book, *How to Talk to Your Kids about Pornography*.

Start the Conversation

Define pornography with the following help. Pornography is pictures or videos of people with little or no clothing. Usually there is sexual behavior in it, but it is always objectification, and it is made for the sole purpose of making money. Help your child understand that objectification is turning a person into a mere thing or object, and choosing to see them without feelings or intelligence.

Explain that it is sometimes used to aid in the sexual abuse of children. Clarify that it is not romantic or at all about love. Describe how it can be addictive. Formulate a plan for what to do if your child sees pornography. Teach them to get away from it, find a trusted adult, and tell a parent. The majority of pornography is now viewed on smart phones and tablets; prepare your child for this probability.

Ask your child if he or she has ever seen pornography. Share your personal or family standards about pornography. Explain that there is nothing wrong with being curious about the human body; curiosity is natural. However pornography is not a healthy way to find answers about the body or sex.

Questions for Your Child

- Have you ever seen pornography? What should you do if you see it?

- Where are some places you might see porn? (While doing homework, on the school bus, at a friend's house, etc.)

- It's good to be curious, but why is looking at pornography to satisfy your curiosity wrong?

- At some point, you will see pornography. What should you do? Who can you tell?

- Will you make a choice and a commitment right now to never seek out pornography?

- What steps can you take to ensure you stick to this commitment?

> *"Stay completely away from pornography. Do not allow yourself to view it, ever. It has been proven to be an addiction which is more than difficult to overcome."*
>
> *—Thomas S. Monson*

Activity

Role play various scenarios where your child is "exposed" to pornography. Model what they can say to a friend or family member who shows them. Discuss what they should do if it pops up on a home or school computer. Have your child take a turn (or several) acting out what they can do if exposed at school, at practice, at church, at a friend's house, etc. Talk about how good kids, who are good friends, may be the ones to show your child porn. Act out how your child can get away from seeing pornography and who they can talk to about it.

Additional Resources:

"Just One Click" from the *Friend*, July 2014

"The Internet is good for lots of things, but sometimes just one click can take you somewhere you don't want to be." –Jessica Larsen

"Crash and Tell" from the *Liahona*, June 2011

This story tells of a boy who accidentally viewed pornography on the family computer, and his mother teaches him about personal revelation. Included are a list of internet safety tips.

"Dads Kill Porn" from Educate and Empower Kids

"[A] dad's warmth and consistent presence appear to have a protective impact on his daughter's sexual development and activity. Conversely, a fatherless daughter may experience sexual development that can far outpace her emotional, social, and neurological development."

"Pornography" from *Gospel Topics*

This page has a lot of information specifically on how to avoid pornography, how to overcome an existing addiction, and more.

24. SEXTING & SOCIAL MEDIA

The research is pouring in, smartphones and social media contribute to depression, anxiety, suicidal ideation, and other mental illnesses in teenagers. Please consider giving your child a phone that does not have internet access (there are several brands now).

Before giving your child a smartphone ask yourself:

- How will my child owning a smartphone contribute to our family's health and happiness?
- How will owning a smartphone help my child to be a kinder, more successful person?
- Does my child really need a phone at school to be successful? (Ask your child's teachers. 90-100% of them will say "no.")

Whether your child has a phone or not, they need to understand the powerful messages in social media and the serious consequences of sexting. Explain to your child that any sexually explicit image or video of a child or teenager is considered child pornography (child abuse sexual material), and that your child can get into serious trouble with school administration and law enforcement for having or sharing these images.

> Sexting:
> The sending or distribution of sexually explicit images, messages, or other material via mobile phones.

Start the Conversation

Go over your household rules for cell phone and social media use. Discuss why these rules benefit everyone and help keep you safe. Consider installing filters and blocks on your computer and child's phone if you have not yet done so. Explain to your children that many kids' first porn exposure happens through social media. Teenagers really should not get any sort of social media account until they are at the very least 13, but hopefully won't be allowed on until they are older.

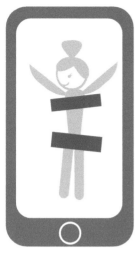

Explain to your child what a sexually explicit text (or sext) is. Discuss what they should do if someone sends them an inappropriate message or sext message. Come up with a plan.

For more information on this, see our free ebook *Social Media and Teens: The Ultimate Guide for Keeping Kids Safe Online*

Questions for Your Child

Q   Social media can be a great tool for people to share uplifting quotes and even to do missionary work. Why do most kids and adults have such a hard time using this technology for good?

Q   Why do so many kids and adults spend hours on social media each day?

Q   Can a person really feel good about themselves after spending an hour or two looking at other people's curated photos and posts?

Q   Who can you talk to if someone asks you for nude photos?

Q   What can you do if someone asks you for a nude photo or picture of your breasts or other parts of your body?

Q   Why is it rude or even sexual harrassment to ask someone for a sexually explicit photo?

Q   Why is it unwise to send a naked picture of yourself?

Additional Resources:

Noah's New Phone: A Story about Using Technology for Good from Educate and Empower Kids

A great family night book featuring a poignant story that addresses smartphone rules, online bullying, social media, and more.

For the Strength of Youth

"Guard your safety and the safety of others by taking great care about what personal information and images you share through technology. Do not communicate anything over the Internet or through texting that would be inappropriate to share in person."

"Teaching Social Media Literacy" from Educate and Empower Kids

"Help your children to understand that the edited photos and exciting lives shown on social media are not an accurate portrayal of their everyday life."

"Talking to Your Kids about Sexting" from Educate and Empower Kids

"Chances are, your child will encounter this at some point in their life, either by unwittingly receiving a sext or feeling pressured to send one or actually sending one. This is why it's so important to talk to our kids about this growing and dangerous trend."

25. BEING MEDIA SAVVY

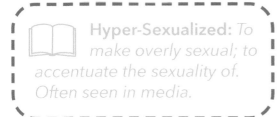

> **Hyper-Sexualized:** *To make overly sexual; to accentuate the sexuality of. Often seen in media.*

Media; we are surrounded by it and heavily influenced by it. For the developing brain of a child, media can profoundly influence how they think of themselves, their bodies, sex, gender, marriage, religion, money, and many other things. Explain to your child how media (TV, movies, pop music, social media, etc.) sends us many unhealthy messages about sex, people, love, and relationships. They must learn to think carefully when choosing media and internalizing its messages.

Teaching our kids to be media literate will not only help them to see through the false and unhealthy messages they are exposed to, it will also help them understand the world around them in a whole new way. Discuss with them the techniques used in video games, online videos, commercials, billboards, etc to create "perfect" looking people, representing a very narrow definition of beauty.

Consider reading our book, *Petra's Power to See: A Media Literacy Adventure*. Your child will learn about media, how to understand its messaging, and how to choose media wisely.

Start the Conversation

Teach your children to question the messages they see in all forms of media, especially messages about sex and love. Ask your kids if they have ever had a negative thought about their body after watching a commercial or video. Discuss ways to counteract the false messages they see every day such as using positive self-talk, knowing the truth about media images, etc. Talk about the fact that commercials are all trying to sell a product and that we should always be looking for the underlying message.

Questions for Your Child

Q What are some TV shows or movies that have good, uplifting messages? What are some shows or YouTube videos that don't have good messages?

Q What are some of the messages we see in TV or movies about love, sex, or relationships? Are these healthy or helpful messages?

Q Why is there so much sexual content and violence in certain shows and movies?

Q What are some of the messages our friends share on social media?

Q How much time should a person spend on a phone or staring at a screen each day?

Q What happens to our mood and overall mental health when we are on screens too much?

> *"And as all have not faith, seek ye diligently and teach one another words of wisdom; yea, seek ye out of the best books words of wisdom, seek learning even by study and also by faith."*
>
> *—Doctrine and Covenants 109:7*

Activity–Deconstructing Media

Watch a commercial with your child and encourage him or her to deconstruct the images and messages within it. Ask your child the following questions:

Q What are your first impressions of this commercial? How did it make you feel?

Q Why was this advertisement made? What was it trying to sell?

Q What values were expressed? What values were not present?

Q Did the actors look like people in our neighborhood?

Q Were the images in the commercial hyper-sexualized or hyper-masculine?

Q After considering the ad this way, how does it make you look at commercials differently?

Additional Resources:

"A Lesson about Media Literacy" from Educate and Empower Kids
"Encourage your child to think about not only the images they see, but the messages that are being presented in the images they see-this is teaching them to deconstruct media."

"A Family's Guide to Digital Media" from Educate and Empower Kids
This free ebook was created to assist you and your family in finding a media balance by providing you the tools and information you need to create your own family media usage plan.

"Choose The Right Media" from the *Friend*, April 2012
This is a guide to help children choose media that is wholesome and uplifting.

"Entertainment and Media" from *For the Strength of Youth*
This section was written specifically to help the youth understand the effects entertainment and media have on their mental and spiritual health.

26. BODY IMAGE

How we feel about our appearance can really affect how we feel about our entire selves. Often we think this is just something that girls and women struggle with, but many men are self-conscious of their looks as well.

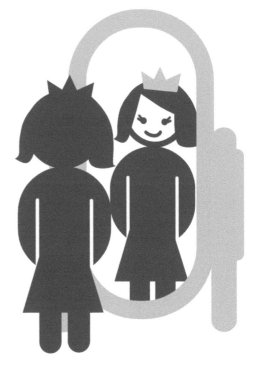

This is a topic that parents need to be particularly wise about as they approach it. You do NOT want to suggest to your child that they specifically will become dissatisfied with their appearance. But your child should know that ALL of us can be highly affected by the many voices around us, whether those are from family members, friends, relatives, movies, social media, etc.

Lesson 25, Being Media Savvy, and our books focusing on healthy body image, _Messages about Me: Sydney's Story, A Girl's Journey to Healthy Body Image_ and _Messages about Me: Wade's Story_, will be very helpful in these discussions. Helping your child to develop a healthy body image will also help improve their overall self-worth!

Start the Conversation

Start by discussing how our culture absurdly places too much emphasis on physical appearance when we have no control over the appearance we were born with. As you talk about healthy body image with your child, explain the importance of accepting and liking one's body just the way it is and striving for real physical health. Talks about ways your family is maintaining good health and what all of you can do to improve your health (meditation, yoga, eating more fruits and vegetables, playing games outside more etc.)

"But the Lord said unto Samuel, Look not on his countenance, or on the height of his stature; because I have refused him: for the Lord seeth not as man seeth; for man looketh on the outward appearance, but the Lord looketh on the heart."

—1 Samuel 16:7

Most importantly, help your child appreciate all their bodies can DO, like jump, sing, learn, laugh, cry, and so much more. Ask your child to name at least 10 things their body can do and then talk about how these things are far more important than one's looks.

Teach your child that they decide their worth, not the media or anybody else. Explain that they will be bombarded by photoshopped, digitized images for the rest of their lives. Because of that, they must learn to look at every image logically. They will need to remind themselves that all media, including social media, are full of fake images with impossible physical standards that no one can attain—not even the people in them. Show your child that they are worthwhile simply because they exist. Behaving in ways that can make them proud of themselves is so much more important than how the world thinks they should look.

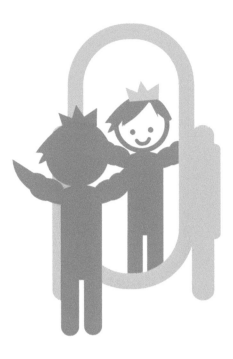

Questions for Your Child

- What do you like about your personality, your abilities, and how your brain works? What do you like about the way you look?
- How does the way you view your body affect the way you feel about yourself as a whole?
- When we spend a lot of time watching TV, YouTube videos, or scrolling through social media, we often compare ourselves to other people. We might feel like everyone else has more stuff than we do or is better looking than us. What can we do to combat these negative feelings?
- Do you think the people on TV look like the people we know in real life?
- Why is being concerned about being a good person more important than worrying about the way we look?
- How might our body image affect how we behave in relationships?

Activity–Share The Love

Have each person in your family share at least two things that he or she likes or loves about every other person in your family. Have one person write down on separate pieces of paper what was said about each family member. Each person must also write down at least two things they like about themselves on this list. Instruct each family member to hang up the list somewhere where they can see it daily.

Tips for Parents

- Remember, your kids are listening to you!
- Stop making negative comments about your body in front of your kids!
- Show your kids your love your body for what it does, not how it looks.
- Teach them to speak kindly to themselves.
- Remind your kids that comparing their bodies to others is not helpful.
- Focus most of your praise on what your kids do, not on their looks.
- If your child struggles with their weight, help them to improve their physical health without emphasizing weight numbers and without making it a moral issue.
- Avoid fashion magazines and hyper-sexualized media in your home.

Additional Resources:

"Confidence and Self-Worth" from the *Ensign*, January 2005

"Let each of us work harder to recognize the accomplishments of others as well as being aware of our own talents and successes. And let us be confident in the knowledge that with the Lord's help, we can accomplish far more than we could ever do on our own." –Glen L. Pace

"My Body Is a Temple" from the *Liahona*, July 2014

"As we care for our bodies the way God has commanded, we will be blessed!" –Marissa Widdison

"Teaching Our Kids about Healthy Body Image" from Educate and Empower Kids

This family night lesson includes great advice to help you teach your child to have a more positive body image.

"Teaching Healthy Body Image to Boys" from Educate and Empower Kids

Includes a lesson for parents that is geared specifically toward helping parents teach their young boys about developing a healthy body image.

27. SELF-WORTH & SELF-ESTEEM

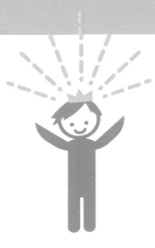

Each and every person is completely unique and special. Our heavenly parents truly love us and have taught and blessed each individual with singular gifts and talents. Help your child understand their worth as a child of God. They are someone who has important work to do here on earth and no one could ever take their place.

Explain to your kids that a person who has healthy self-worth behaves differently from someone who does not. A person who is proud of themselves and can admire their own behavior will NOT do or ask others to do things that make them uncomfortable.

Our book _30 Days to a Stronger Child_ is a great resource with amazing family night discussions on self-confidence, empathy, assertiveness, positive self-talk, as well as other topics related to our intellectual, spiritual, physical, social, and emotional health.

Start the Conversation

Help separate your child's appearance from his or her self-worth. Describe some of the actions a person who doesn't feel good about themselves might take: he might be sad, she might tease others, he might hide his body, she might show too much of her body to get attention, etc. A person with self-respect is confident, kind, and won't do anything intentionally to hurt others or make them feel uncomfortable. Ask your child how a person's dress, demeanor, facial expressions, language, and actions are reflections of how they feel about themselves. Most importantly, teach your child that comparing themselves to others is unproductive and does not lead to true self-worth!

Questions for Your Child

- Q There is no one else in the whole universe that is the same as you. Why did God ensure each of us was different and special?
- Q How are you special to God? How are you special to our family?
- Q What are your skills and talents?

- Each of us has spiritual gifts; what might be one of your missions here on earth? What can you do to make the world a better place?
- How might a person who feels good about him or herself act differently from someone who does not?
- Where do you find your worth? What qualities do you admire in yourself?
- How does one's self-worth affect the way they treat others?
- How might self-worth affect ones decision to enter a relationship or have sex?

"She is more precious than rubies: and all the things thou canst desire are not to be compared unto her."

—Proverbs 3:15

Activity—You are Unique and Special

Make a list of all the things you can think of that make YOU wonderful inside and out. Think about the unique way you sleep, eat, walk, run, do homework, make friends, play games, talk with others, write stories, etc. Think about your unique tastes in books, movies, friends, foods, and whatever else you like. What makes you YOU? Have each member of your family make a list and then share them with one another.

Additional Resources:

"Young Women Theme"
"I am a beloved daughter of heavenly parents, with a divine nature and eternal destiny."

"Aaronic Priesthood Theme"
"I am a beloved son of God, and He has a work for me to do."

"Learning Positive Self-Talk" from Educate and Empower Kids
"Children must learn their self-worth should be based on who they are intrinsically, instead of their ability to fit into popular culture."

"What You're Worth and How to Know It" from the New Era, July 2017
"Our divine worth is constant—and it comes from who we are: divine children of a loving Heavenly Father with the potential to become like Him." –Hadley Griggs

"5 Ways a Mother Can Develop Self-Worth in Her Son" from Educate and Empower Kids
This article offers mothers a variety of ways that they can help their sons to develop positive self-worth.

"5 Things a Father Can Do to Increase His Daughter's Self-Worth" from Educate and Empower Kids
This article describes a number of ways that fathers can help their daughters to develop positive self-worth.

28. SHAME & GUILT

Helping kids understand the difference between shame and guilt is something that will not only help them in their sexual education, but in their spiritual education as well. Remember, guilt is the idea, "I made a mistake." Shame is the idea, "I am a terrible person." Guilt can lead to repentance, making amends, and creating lasting change in our lives. This is a great opportunity to discuss how repentance is always positive.

> *"The Spirit's voice will never encourage you to hate yourself, rather reminding you of your eternal worth as a child of God (see Moses 1:4). The voice that says you are worthless and unlovable will always be Satan's (see Moses 1:12)."*
>
> —McKell A. Jorgensen, Jan. 2020 *Ensign*

Point out that some people think sex is bad or dirty. Teach your children that this is a sad myth. Sex is not bad. It is wonderful and healthy! God gave us these powerful procreative powers. However, some people feel embarrassed about it, so they make others feel guilty or ashamed about it as well. Remind your kids that sex is a normal, natural act for adults.

Start the Conversation

Sexual intercourse is a very intimate act that often happens naked, which makes people feel vulnerable, sometimes leading to feelings of guilt and shame. Explain the difference between guilt and shame. Ask your child what situations could cause shame about sex.

Use the glossary to discuss consent and sexual assault. Help your child understand that sexual assault is against the law and that the abuser should feel terrible for what they've done, and needs to be punished accordingly. However, sexual assault often causes the victim to feel shame and guilt, but an assault is NEVER the victim's fault! Teach your child that if anything abusive ever happens to them, they need not feel ashamed.

Questions for Your Child

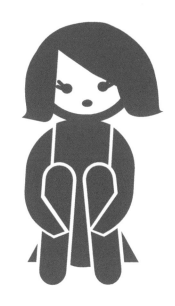

- Why is guilt a good thing? (It is the Holy Ghost prompting us to make a change.)
- What is the difference between guilt and shame?
- When we have made a mistake or sinned, how can we stop ourselves from feeling shame and instead focus on what we can do to make things better and move forward?
- God never uses shame, not even when we have sinned. Why does Satan use shame?
- Sometimes kids and adults who have been sexually abused feel shame or blame themselves for what was done to them. Why do you think this happens?
- What have you learned about sex that can help you to have a positive attitude toward it?
- Why do some people feel shameful or guilty about sex?
- What can you do if you feel guilty or ashamed about something you have done or seen?

Additional Resources:

"The Biggest Barrier to Our Connection with God" from *Inspiration*, January 2018

"Trusting deep down that you are loved by an eternal father is also the key to believing you are worthy of connecting with Him all the time, even when you mess up." –Celeste Davis

"Three Mistakes I've Made Using Shame and Guilt" from Educate and Empower Kids

This article describes some of the ways parents may inadvertently teach their children to associate shame and guilt with body image and behavior.

"Teaching Without Shame: Understanding Your Child's Curiosity" from Educate and Empower Kids

This article teaches how to talk to your kids about their natural curiosity and how to instruct without making them feel ashamed of themselves.

"Eight Myths about Repentance" from the *New Era*, March 2016

This article goes through a few misconceptions about repentance and tries to help readers understand more about what the process actually is.

"Shame versus Guilt: Help for Discerning God's Voice from Satan's Lies" from the *Ensign*, January 2020

This article does a great job at helping define the difference between shame and guilt, and it helps readers to understand how these two feelings work in relation to repentance.

29. PREGNANCY

Describe conception and pregnancy. As you discuss these, add any additional information you think your child may need. This may also be a good time to discuss infertility, adoption, and abortion. Feel free to discuss your cultural and spiritual beliefs in regards to pregnancy and birth control. You may feel prompted to talk about why the Church condemns abortion unless the pregnancy is the result of incest or rape, or when the life or health of the mother is in danger.

Check the glossary for any definitions you may need such as uterus, vagina, penis, fertilize, gestation, abstinence, contraceptive, the pill, condom, etc.

Start the Conversation

Explain to your child that although sex is usually required for someone to get pregnant, one does not become pregnant every time she has sex. Although seemingly commonplace and "natural," the act of reproduction represents somewhat of a miracle in the creation of a new organism. Since it only takes one sperm to fertilize an egg, pregnancy can occur even if there is no ejaculation. Any vaginal, sexual intercourse can cause a pregnancy.

Then explain how conception works: When a man ejaculates, millions of sperm are propelled into the vagina. From there, the sperm must swim through the vagina and the cervix and up the fallopian tube. Only a few dozen sperm may actually make it to the egg. The fastest and strongest sperm can make the trip in around 45 minutes, but fertilization can occur up to a week after sex. Once the sperm reaches the egg, there is a frantic effort to get through the cell wall. The first one in causes a cellular reaction making the fertilized egg impenetrable to any other sperm. The fertilized egg is now an embryo. At the instant of fertilization, the baby's genes and sex are set. If the sperm has a Y chromosome, your baby will be a boy. If it has an X chromosome, the baby will be a girl.

The fertilized egg stays in the fallopian tube for about 3 to 4 days, but within 24 hours of being fertilized, it quickly starts dividing into many cells. It keeps dividing as it moves slowly through the fallopian tube to the uterus. Its next job is to attach to the lining of the uterus. This is called implantation. During pregnancy, the embryo or fetus grows and develops inside a woman's uterus. A full-term pregnancy lasts approximately 40 weeks.

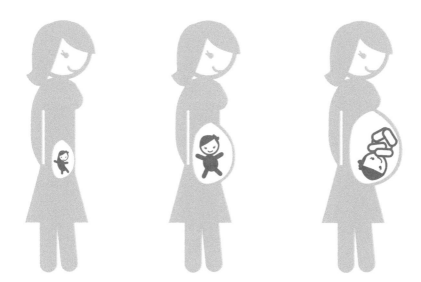

 If no sperm is around to fertilize the egg, it passes through to the uterus and disintegrates. A woman's hormone levels then go back to normal and her body sheds the thick lining of the uterus, and her period starts.

Questions for Your Child

Q What other physical changes happen to a woman's body during pregnancy?

Q Do you know how to prevent pregnancy?

Q Pregnancies can be difficult and painful. Why would women choose to have a baby?

Q Some people refer to pregnancy as co-creating with God. What does this mean?

Q What are the blessings that come from having a child?

Q Are there advantages to a child who is born in a family with two committed, married parents?

Q Why is the family "ordained of God"?

Q Let's review lesson #7, do you remember how a woman becomes pregnant?

"Our birth is but a sleep
and a forgetting;/
The Soul that rises with us,
our life's Star/ . . .
But trailing clouds of glory
do we come/
From God, who is our home:/"

—William Wordsworth

Activity

Talk about some of the funny, strange, and difficult experiences with yours or your spouse's pregnancy. Explain some of the joy, fear, and wonder you felt at carrying and giving birth to a child. Show your child photos or videos of the day they were born. Express your love and gratitude that God sent your child to your family.

Ask your child the following questions:

- Do you want to be a parent someday? Why or Why not?
- How many children would you like to have someday?
- What do you imagine pregnancy will be like for you (or your spouse)?
- Many people are not able to have children on their own. What can a couple do if they are not able to physically have children? (Discuss adoption and fertility options.)

Additional Resources:

"The Lord's standard regarding sexual purity is clear and unchanging. Do not have any sexual relations before marriage, and be completely faithful to your spouse after marriage . . . In God's sight, sexual sins are extremely serious. They defile the sacred power God has given us to create life." -For the Strength of Youth

"Teaching about Procreation and Chastity"

We are all children of God with biological parents and heavenly parents.

"Talking with Your Children about Moral Purity" from the Ensign, December 1986

"We may want to describe the peace and confidence that fidelity brings to our marriage relationship and, on the contrary, what infidelity does to destroy homes and families."

"4 Easy Steps to Creating Healthy Communication about Sexual Intimacy" from Educate and Empower Kids

"When we make it clear to our children that we will talk to them about anything-no boundaries-we encourage them to come to us, rather than plunging down the wormhole of the internet."

30. STDs & STIs

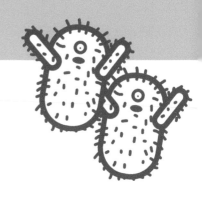

There are many kinds of sexually transmitted diseases (STDs) and sexually transmitted infections (STIs). Use the glossary to help you discuss some or all of these with your kids. Be specific and teach your children how these can be spread through vaginal, anal, and oral sex. (See the glossary for definitions.)

Teach your kids how to prevent STDs and STIs, and discuss how one can find out if they have been infected and where one could get tested.

> **STD:** *An abbreviation that refers to sexually transmitted diseases. These are illnesses that are communicable through sexual behaviors, including intercourse. Some of these illnesses can also be transmitted through blood contact.*

Start the Conversation

Ask your child if they have heard of AIDS, HIV, HPV, herpes, syphilis, hepatitis B or C, chlamydia, pubic lice, and/or gonorrhea. Use the glossary to help you define these. Explain that these are all sexually transmitted infections or diseases and that some of them are deadly. Others won't kill, but will stay in the body for life.

Talk about the best ways to avoid STIs and STDs, like abstinence, monogamy, and condom use. Many people have begun transitioning from using the term STD to using STI in an effort to clarify that not all sexually transmitted infections turn into a disease.

Questions for Your Child

Q What are sexually transmitted diseases (STDs) and sexually transmitted infections (STIs)? Do you understand how they are spread?

Q Why are these diseases harmful? Which ones are incurable?

Q How does avoiding sex until marriage keep you safe from STDs?

- What other reasons do we have for waiting until marriage to have sex?
- How are diseases and infections spread? How are STDs and STIs different from colds, flu, warts, and other illnesses? (These other illnesses are spread through human contact and bodily fluid, but STIs and STDs are transmitted through sexual contact with an infected person.)

> *"And go ye out from among the wicked. Save yourselves. Be ye clean that bear the vessels of the Lord."*
>
> *–Doctrine and Covenants 38:42*

Additional Resources:

Church Policies and Guidelines

"Members who are infected with HIV (human immunodeficiency virus) or who have AIDS (acquired immunodeficiency syndrome) should be welcomed at Church meetings and activities."

"Talking with Your Children about Moral Purity" from the *Ensign*, December 1986

"One reason we live the law of chastity is to show that we love God and are obedient to his law. Avoiding unwed pregnancy and the diseases that are sometimes transmitted by sexual contact are other good reasons for being chaste, but even more important are the great blessings of self-respect, a clear conscience, the companionship of the Holy Ghost, self-control, being trusted, and being worthy of a mission and temple marriage. Each of these blessings is worthy of a parent-child discussion."

"Lead Me, Guide Me" from the *New Era*, November 2001

Many of us will face unwanted or unexpected illnesses. This article talks about how no matter what, God loves you and the Holy Ghost will always be there to comfort you.

"Why Me?" from the *New Era*, December 2009

This article talks of the trials of illness and disease, and that the Lord will always be by our side whenever the storms of life hit us.

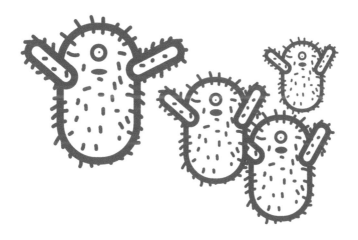

GLOSSARY

The following terms have been included to assist you as you prepare and hold discussions with your children regarding healthy sexuality and intimacy. The definitions are not intended for the child; rather, they are meant to clarify the concepts and terms for the adult. Some terms may not be appropriate for your child, given their age, circumstances, or your own family culture and values. Use your judgment to determine which terminology best meets your individual needs.

Abortion: An abortion is a procedure to end a pregnancy. It uses medicine and/or surgery to remove the embryo or fetus and placenta from the uterus.

Abstinence: The practice of not doing or having something that is wanted or enjoyable; the practice of abstaining from something.

Abuse: The improper usage or treatment of another person or entity, often to unfairly gain power and/or other benefit in the relationship.

Affection: A feeling of liking or caring for something or someone. A type of love that surpasses general goodwill.

AIDS: A sexually transmitted or blood-borne viral infection that causes immune deficiency.

Anal Sex: A form of intercourse that generally involves the insertion and thrusting of the erect penis into the anus and rectum for sexual pleasure.

Anus: The external opening of the rectum, composed of two sphincters which control the exit of feces from the body.

Appropriate: Suitable, proper, or fitting for a particular purpose, person, or circumstance.

Arousal (in regards to sexual activities): The physical and emotional response to sexual desire during or in anticipation of sexual activity. In men, this results in an erection. In women, this results in vaginal lubrication (wetness) and engorgement of the clitoris and vaginal walls.

Birth Control: The practice of preventing unwanted pregnancies, especially by use of contraception. See also IUD, condom, contraceptive implant, and the pill.

Birth Control Shot: Commonly referred to as the birth control shot, Depo-Provera® is an injectable form of birth control. This contraceptive option is a shot that contains the hormone progesterone and is given on a regular schedule.

Bisexual: A sexual orientation in which one is attracted to both males and females.

Body Image: An individual's feelings regarding their own physical appearance, attractiveness and/or sexuality. These feelings and opinions are often influenced by other people and media sources.

Bodily Integrity: The personal belief that our bodies, while crucial to our understanding of who we are, do not in themselves solely define our worth. The knowledge that our bodies are the storehouse of our humanity, and the sense that we esteem our bodies and we treat them accordingly. It is also defined as the right to autonomy and self-determination over one's own body.

Boundaries: The personal limits or guidelines that an individual forms in order to clearly identify what are reasonable and safe behaviors for others to engage in around him or her.

Bowel Movement: Also known as defecation, a bowel movement is the final act of digestion by which waste is eliminated from the body via the anus.

Breasts: Breasts contain mammary glands, which create the breast milk used to feed infants. Women develop breasts on their upper torso during puberty.

Child: A term often used in reference to individuals who are under the age of 18. This overlaps with the term, teen.

Circumcision: The surgical removal of foreskin from a baby's penis.

Chlamydia: A common sexually transmitted infection caused by the bacteria chlamydia trachomatis. It can affect the eyes and may cause damage to a woman's reproductive system.

Clitoris: A female sex organ visible at the front juncture of the labia minora above the opening of the urethra. The clitoris is the female's most sensitive erogenous zone.

Condom: A thin rubber covering that a man wears on his penis during sex in order to prevent a woman from becoming pregnant and/or to help prevent the spread of diseases.

Consent: Clear agreement or permission to permit something or to do something. Consent must be given freely, without force or intimidation, while the person is fully conscious and cognizant of their present situation.

Contraceptive: A method, device, or medication that works to prevent pregnancy. Another name for birth control. See birth control, IUD, condom, or diaphragm.

Contraceptive Implant: Contraceptive implants are a long-term birth control option for women. A contraceptive implant is a flexible plastic rod about the size of a matchstick that is placed under the skin of the upper arm.

Curiosity: The desire to learn or know more about something or someone.

Date Rape: A rape that is committed by someone with a person they have gone on a date with. The perpetrator uses physical force, psychological intimidation, and/or drugs or alcohol to force the victim to have sex either against their will or in a state in which they cannot give clear consent.

Degrade: To treat with contempt or disrespect.

Demean: To cause a severe loss in dignity or respect in another person.

Derogatory: An adjective that implies severe criticism or loss of respect.

Diaphragm (Contraceptive): A cervical barrier type of birth control made of a soft latex or silicone dome with a spring molded into the rim. The spring creates a seal against the walls of the vagina, preventing semen, including sperm, from entering the fallopian tubes.

Domestic Abuse/Domestic Violence: A pattern of abusive behavior in any relationship that is used by one partner to gain and/or maintain power and control over another in a domestic setting. It can be physical, sexual, emotional, economic, and/or psychological actions or threats of actions that harm another person. (from the Department of Justice)

Double Standard: A rule or standard that is applied differently and/or unfairly to a person or distinct groups of people.

Egg Cell: The female reproductive cell, which, when fertilized by sperm, will eventually grow into an infant.

Ejaculation: When a man reaches orgasm, semen is expelled from the penis.

Emotion: An emotion is a feeling such as happiness, love, fear, sadness, or anger, which can be caused by the situation that you are in or the people you are with.

Emotional Abuse: A form of abuse in which another person is subjected to behavior that can result in psychological trauma. Emotional abuse often occurs within relationships where there is a power imbalance.

Emotional Intimacy: A form of intimacy that displays a degree of closeness which focuses more on the emotional over the physical aspects of a relationship.

Epididymal Hypertension: A condition that results from prolonged sexual arousal in human males in which fluid congestion in the testicles occurs, often accompanied by testicular pain. The condition is temporary, and is also referred to as "blue balls."

Erection: When the penis becomes engorged/enlarged with blood, often as a result of sexual arousal.

Explicit: In reference to sexual content, "sexually explicit" is meant to signify that the content with such a warning will portray sexual content openly and clearly to the viewers.

Extortion: To obtain something through force or threats, particularly sex or money.

Family: A group consisting of parents and children living together in a household. The definition of family is constantly evolving, and every person can define family in a different way to encompass the relationships he or she shares with people in his or her life. Over time one's family will change as one's life changes and the importance of family values and rituals deepen.

Female Arousal: The physiological responses to sexual desire during or in anticipation of sexual activity in women. This includes vaginal lubrication (wetness), engorgement of the external genitals (clitoris and labia), enlargement of the vagina, and dilation of the pupils.

Fertilize: The successful union between an egg (ovum) and a sperm, which normally occurs within the second portion of the fallopian tube, also known as the ampulla. The result of fertilization is a zygote (fertilized egg).

Forced Affection: Pressuring or forcing a child to give a hug, kiss, or any other form of physical affection when they do not have the desire to do so.

Foreskin: The fold of skin which covers the head (the glans) of the penis. Also called the prepuce.

Friend: Someone with whom a person has a relationship of mutual affection and is typically closer than an associate or acquaintance.

Gay: A slang term used to describe people who are sexually attracted to members of the same sex. The term "lesbian" is generally used when talking about women who are attracted to other women. Originally, the word "gay" meant "carefree;" its connection to sexual orientation developed during the latter half of the 20th century.

Gender: Masculinity and femininity are differentiated through a range of characteristics known as "gender." However, use of this term may include biological sex (being male or female), social roles based upon biological sex, and/or one's subjective experience and understanding of their own gender identity.

Gender Role: The commonly perceived pattern of masculine or feminine behavior as defined by an individual's culture and/or upbringing.

Gender Stereotypes: A generalized thought or understanding applied to either males or females (or other gender identities) that may or may not correspond with reality. "Men don't cry" or "women are weak" are examples of inaccurate gender stereotypes.

Gestation: The period of time when a person or animal is developing inside its mother's womb preparing to be born.

Gonorrhea: A sexually transmitted disease that affects both males and females, usually in the rectum, throat, and/or urethra. It can also infect the cervix in females.

Grooming (Predatory): To prepare/train and/or desensitize someone, usually a child, with the intent of committing a sexual offense and/or harm.

Healthy Sexuality: Having the ability to express one's sexuality in ways that contribute positively to one's own self-esteem and relationships. Healthy sexuality includes approaching sexual relationships and interactions with mutual agreement and dignity. It must include mutual respect and a lack of fear, shame, or guilt, and never includes coercion or violence.

Hepatitis B: Hepatitis B (HBV) is an incurable disease which is most commonly spread through exposure to infected bodily fluids via unclean needles, unscreened blood, and/or sexual content. It can manifest as acute or chronic. The acute form can resolve itself in less than six months, but it will often turn chronic. The chronic form can persist in the body for a lifetime and lead to a number of serious illnesses including cirrhosis and liver cancer. The younger a person is exposed to HBV, the more likely it will become chronic.

Hepatitis C: Transmitted in a similar manner to Hepatitis B, Hepatitis C attacks the liver. Though most individuals with Hepatitis C are asymptomatic, individuals who do develop symptoms typically show signs of yellowing skin and eyes, fatigue, and/or nausea.

Herpes: A series of diseases of the skin caused by the herpes virus which cause sores and inflammation of the skin. Type 1 viruses will manifest as cold sores on the lips or nose, while the type 2 viruses are sexually transmitted and specifically known as genital herpes. This causes painful sores on the genital area.

Heterosexual: Sexual orientation in which one is attracted to members of the opposite sex (males are attracted to females; females are attracted to males). See also, straight.

HIV: HIV (human immunodeficiency virus) is a virus that attacks the body's immune system. If not treated, it will turn into AIDS. It is incurable and will persist in the body for life. It is spread through infected bodily fluids and sexual contact.

Homosexual: Sexual orientation in which one is attracted to members of the same sex (males are attracted to males; females are attracted to females). See also gay or lesbian.

Hook-up Sex: A form of casual sex in which sexual activity takes place outside the context of a committed relationship. The sex may be a one-time event, or an ongoing arrangement. In either case, the focus is generally on the physical enjoyment of sexual activity without an emotional involvement or commitment.

HPV: Human papillomavirus. It is the most common STD in the United States and can cause genital warts or cancer in about 10% of those infected. Anyone over age 10 can receive the vaccine for HPV.

Hymen: A membrane that partially closes the opening of the vagina and whose presence is traditionally taken to be a mark of virginity. However, it can often be broken before a woman has sex simply by being active, and sometimes it is not present at all.

Hyper-sexualized: To make extremely sexual; to emphasize the sexuality of. Often seen in media.

Instinct: An inherent response or inclination toward a particular behavior. An action or reaction that is performed without being based on prior experience.

Intercourse: Sexual activity, also known as coitus or copulation, that is most commonly understood to refer to the insertion of the penis into the vagina (vaginal sex). It should be noted that there are a wide range of various sexual activities and the boundaries of what constitutes sexual intercourse are still under debate. See also, sex.

Intersex: An umbrella term used to refer to the rare phenomenon of an individual born with some mixture of both male and female reproductive anatomy. This can be very obvious with visibly deformed or underdeveloped reproductive organs, to something as subtle as alterations in the XY chromosomes. It's also possible for signs of intersex to not develop until later in life.

Intimacy: Generally, a feeling or form of significant closeness. There are four types of intimacy: physical intimacy (sensual proximity or touching), emotional intimacy (close connection resulting from trust and love), cognitive or intellectual intimacy (resulting from honest exchange of thoughts and ideas), and experiential intimacy (a connection that occurs while working together). Emotional and physical intimacy are often associated with sexual relationships, while intellectual and experiential intimacy are not. However, people can engage in a sexual experience that is devoid of intimacy.

IUD: A small, T-shaped device that is placed in the uterus to prevent pregnancy.

Labia: The inner and outer folds of the vulva on both sides of the vagina.

Lesbian: A word used to describe women who are sexually attracted to other women.

Lice (Pubic): A sexually transmitted sucking louse infesting the pubic region of the human body.

Love: A wide range of emotional interpersonal connections, feelings, and attitudes. Common forms include kinship or familial love, friendship, divine love (as demonstrated through worship), and sexual or romantic love. In biological terms, love is the attraction and bonding that functions to unite human beings and facilitate the social and sexual continuation of the species.

Masturbation: Self-stimulation of the genitals in order to produce sexual arousal, pleasure, and/or orgasm.

Media Literacy: The ability to study, interpret, and create messages in various media such as books, social media posts, online ads, movies, etc. It also includes understanding how to navigate being online, what to avoid, and what information to share and/or keep private.

Menstrual Cycle: The egg is released from ovaries through the fallopian tube into the uterus. Each month, a lining of blood and tissue build up in the uterus. When the egg is not fertilized, this lining is no longer needed and is shed from the body through the vagina. The cycle is roughly 28 days, but can vary between individuals. The bleeding lasts around 2-7 days. The menstrual cycle may be accompanied by cramping, breast tenderness, and emotional sensitivity.

Menstrual Period: A discharging of blood, secretions, and tissue debris from the uterus as it sheds its thickened lining (endometrium) approximately once per month in females who've reached a fertile age. This does not occur during pregnancy.

Misandry: Like misogyny, it is the hatred, aversion, hostility, or dislike of men or boys. Similarly, it also can appear in a single individual, or may also be manifest in broad cultural trends.

Misogyny: The hatred, aversion, hostility, or dislike of women or girls. Misogyny can appear in a single individual, or may also be manifest in broad cultural trends that undermine women's autonomy and value.

Molestation: Aggressive and persistent harassment, either psychological or physical, of a sexual manner.

Monogamy: A relationship in which a person has one partner at any one time.

Nipples: The circular, somewhat conical structure of tissue on the breast. The skin of the nipple and its surrounding areola are often several shades darker than that of the surrounding breast tissue. In women, the nipple delivers breast milk to infants.

Nocturnal Emissions: A spontaneous orgasm that occurs during sleep. Nocturnal emissions can occur in both males (ejaculation) and females (lubrication of the vagina). The term "wet dream" is often used to describe male nocturnal emissions.

Non-binary/Genderqueer: Non-binary or genderqueer is an umbrella term for gender identities that are neither male nor female—identities that are outside the gender binary. Non-binary identities fall under the transgender umbrella, since non-binary people typically identify with a gender that is different from their assigned sex.

Nudity: The state of not wearing any clothing. Full nudity denotes a complete absence of clothing, while partial nudity is a more ambiguous term, denoting the presence of an indeterminate amount of clothing.

Oral Sex: Sexual activity that involves stimulation of the genitals through the use of another person's mouth.

Orgasm: The rhythmic muscular contractions in the pelvic region that occur as a result of sexual stimulation, arousal, and activity during the sexual response cycle. Orgasms are characterized by a sudden release of built-up sexual tension and the resulting sexual pleasure.

Penis: The external, male sexual organ comprised of the shaft, foreskin, glans penis, and meatus. The penis contains the urethra, through which both urine and semen travel to exit the body.

Perception: A way of regarding, understanding, or interpreting something; a mental impression.

Period: The beginning of the menstrual cycle.

Physical Abuse: The improper physical treatment of another person with the intent to cause bodily harm, pain, or other suffering. Physical abuse is often employed to unfairly gain power or other benefit in the relationship.

The Pill: An oral contraceptive for women containing the hormones estrogen and progesterone or progesterone alone. This prevents ovulation, fertilization, or implantation of a fertilized ovum, causing temporary infertility.

Polyamory: The practice of engaging in multiple romantic (and typically sexual) relationships, with the agreement of all the people involved.

Pornography: The portrayal of explicit sexual content for the purpose of causing sexual arousal. In it, sex and bodies are commodified for the purpose of making a financial profit. It can be created in a variety of media contexts, including videos, photos, animation, books and magazines. Its most lucrative means of distribution is through the internet. The industry that creates pornography is a sophisticated, corporatized, billion-dollar business.

Positive Self-Talk: Anything said to oneself for encouragement or motivation, such as phrases or mantras; also, one's ongoing internal conversation with oneself, like a running commentary, which influences how one feels and behaves.

(Sexual) Predator: A sexual predator is someone who seeks to obtain sexual contact/pleasure from another through predatory and/or abusive behavior. The term is often used to describe the deceptive and coercive methods used by people who commit sex crimes where there is a victim.

Pregnancy: The common term used for gestation in humans. During pregnancy, the embryo or fetus grows and develops inside a woman's uterus.

Premature Ejaculation: When a man regularly reaches orgasm, during which semen is expelled from the penis, prior to or within one minute of the initiation of sexual activity.

Priapism: The technical term of a condition in which the erect penis does not return to flaccidity within four hours, despite the absence of physical or psychological sexual stimulation.

Private: Belonging to or for the use of a specific individual. Private and privacy denote a state of being alone, solitary, individual, exclusive, secret, personal, hidden, and confidential.

Psychological Abuse: A form of abuse where the abuser regularly uses a range of actions or words with the intent to manipulate, weaken, or confuse a person's thoughts. This distorts the victim's sense of self and harms their mental wellbeing. Psychological abuse often occurs within relationships in which there is a power imbalance.

Puberty: A period or process through which children reach sexual maturity. Once a person has reached puberty, their body is capable of sexual reproduction.

Public: Belonging to or for the use of all people in a specific area, or all people as a whole. Something that is public is common, shared, collective, communal, and widespread.

Queer: A historically derogatory term against people who were homosexual, that has been reclaimed by the LGBTQ+ community. It is also an umbrella term for sexual and gender minorities who are not heterosexual.

Rape: A sex crime in which the perpetrator forces another person to have sexual intercourse against their will and without consent. Rape often occurs through the threat or actuality of violence against the victim.

Rape Culture: A culture in which rape is pervasive and, to an extent, normalized due to cultural and societal attitudes toward gender and sexuality. Behaviors that facilitate rape culture include victim blaming, sexual objectification, and denial regarding sexual violence.

Relationship: The state of being connected, united, or related to another person.

Rhythm Method: A method of avoiding pregnancy by restricting sexual intercourse to the times of a woman's menstrual cycle when ovulation and conception are least likely to occur. Because it can be difficult to predict ovulation, the effectiveness of the rhythm method is on average just 75–87%.

Romantic Love: A form of love that denotes intimacy and a strong desire for emotional connection with another person to whom one is generally also sexually attracted.

Scrotum: The pouch of skin underneath the penis that contains the testicles.

Self-Worth/Self-Esteem: An individual's overall emotional evaluation of their own worth. Self-worth is both a judgment of the self and an attitude toward the self. More generally, the term is used to describe a confidence in one's own value or abilities.

Semen: The male reproductive fluid, which contains spermatozoa in suspension. Semen exits the penis through ejaculation.

Serial Monogamy: A mating system in which a man or woman can only form a long-term, committed relationship (such as marriage) with one partner at a time. Should the relationship dissolve, the individual may go on to form another relationship, but only after the first relationship has ceased.

Sex (Sexual Intercourse): Sexual activity, also known as coitus or copulation, which is most commonly understood to refer to the insertion of the penis into the vagina (vaginal sex). It should be noted that there are a wide range of various sexual activities and the boundaries of what constitutes sexual intercourse are still under debate. See also, intercourse.

Sexting: The sending or distribution of sexually explicit images, messages, or other material via phones, email, or instant messaging.

Sexual Abuse: The improper sexual usage or treatment of another person, often to unfairly gain power or other benefit in the relationship. In instances of sexual abuse, undesired sexual behaviors are forced upon one person by another.

Sexual Assault: A term often used in legal contexts to refer to sexual violence. Sexual assault occurs when there is any non-consensual sexual contact or violence. Examples include rape, groping, forced kissing, child sexual abuse, and sexual torture.

Sexual Harassment: Harassment involving unwanted sexual advances or obscene remarks. Sexual harassment can be a form of sexual coercion as well as an undesired sexual proposition, including the promise of reward in exchange for sexual favors.

Sexual Identification: How one thinks of oneself in terms of whom one is romantically or sexually attracted to.

Shame: The painful feeling arising from the consciousness of something dishonorable, improper, ridiculous, etc., done by oneself or another.

Slut-shaming: The act of criticizing, attacking, or shaming a woman for her real or presumed sexual activity, or for behaving in ways that someone thinks are associated with her real or presumed sexual activity.

Sperm: The male reproductive cell, consisting of a head, midpiece, and tail. The head contains the genetic material, while the tail is used to propel the sperm as it travels towards the egg.

Spontaneous Erection: A penile erection that occurs as an automatic response to a variety of stimuli, some of which is sexual and some of which is physiological.

STD: An abbreviation that refers to sexually transmitted diseases, many of which persist in the body for life. These are illnesses that are communicable through sexual behaviors, including intercourse. Some of these illnesses can also be transmitted through contact with various bodily fluids.

STI: An abbreviation that refers to sexually transmitted infections. These are illnesses that are communicable through sexual behaviors, including intercourse. Some of these illnesses can be transmitted through blood contact. Not all STI's lead to a disease and become an STD.

Straight: A slang term for heterosexuality, a sexual orientation in which one is attracted to members of the opposite sex (males are attracted to females; females are attracted to males). See also, heterosexual.

Syphilis: Syphilis is an infection typically spread through sexual contact. It is a chronic, contagious, usually venereal and often congenital disease. If left untreated, syphilis can produce chancres, rashes, and systemic lesions in a clinical course with three stages continued over many years.

Test Touch: Seemingly innocent touches by a predator or offender, such as a pat on the back or a squeeze on the arm, that are meant to normalize kids to being in physical contact with the predator. Test touches can quickly progress from these innocent touches to more dangerous and damaging ones.

Testicles: The male gonad, which is located inside the scrotum beneath the penis. The testicles are responsible for the production of sperm and androgens, primarily testosterone.

Transgender: A condition or state in which one's physical sex does not match one's perceived gender identity. A transgender individual may have been assigned a sex at birth based on their genitals, but feel that this assignation is false or incomplete. They also may be someone who does not wish to be identified by conventional gender roles and instead combines or moves between them (often referred to as gender-fluid).

Uncomfortable: Feeling or causing discomfort or unease; disquieting.

Under the Influence: Being physically affected by alcohol or drugs.

Urethra: The tube that connects the urinary bladder to the urinary meatus (the orifice through which the urine exits the urethra tube). In males, the urethra runs down the penis and opens at the end of the penis. In females, the urethra is internal and opens between the clitoris and the vagina.

Urination: The process through which urine is released from the urinary bladder to travel down the urethra and exit the body at the urinary meatus.

Uterus: A major reproductive sex organ in the female body. The uterus is located in the lower half of the torso, just above the vagina. It is the site in which offspring are conceived and in which they gestate during pregnancy.

Vagina: The muscular tube leading from the external genitals to the cervix of the uterus in women. During sexual intercourse, the penis can be inserted into the vagina. During childbirth, the infant exits the uterus through the vagina.

Vaginal Discharge/Secretions: Vaginal discharge is the umbrella term for the clear/milky white fluid that secretes from the vagina daily. This discharge is the means by which the vagina keeps itself clean by discharging cells and debris. When a woman is sexually aroused, she will see an increase in this secretion as a means of preparing the vagina for sex.

Vaginal Sex: A form of sexual intercourse in which the penis is inserted into the vagina.

Vaginismus: A medical condition in which a woman experiences pain from any form of vaginal penetration, including sexual intercourse, the use of tampons or menstrual cups, and/or gynecological examinations.

Victim: A person who is harmed, injured, or killed as the result of an accident or crime.

Virgin: A person, male or female, who has never engaged in sexual intercourse.

Vulva: The parts of the female sexual organs that are on the outside of the body.

Wet Dreams: A slang term for nocturnal emissions. A nocturnal emission is a spontaneous orgasm that occurs during sleep. Nocturnal emissions can occur in both males (ejaculation) and females (lubrication of the vagina).

NOTES

Notes:

Notes:

Notes: